Accident & Emergency Radiology

A SURVIVAL GUIDE

Third Edition

Nigel Raby, MB ChB, MRCP, FRCR
Consultant Radiologist, Western Infirmary, Glasgow

Laurence Berman, MB BS, FRCP, FRCR
Lecturer and Honorary Consultant Radiologist,
University of Cambridge and Addenbrooke's Hospital, Cambridge

Simon Morley, MA, BM BCh, MRCP, FRCR
Consultant Radiologist, University College Hospitals, London

Gerald de Lacey, MA, MB BChir, FRCR
Consultant to Radiology Red Dot Courses, London
(www.radiology-courses.com)

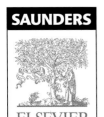

SAUNDERS

ELSEVIER

Edinburgh • London • New York • Oxford • Philad
St Louis • Sydney • Toronto 2015

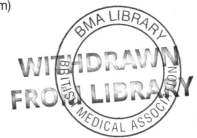

SAUNDERS an imprint of Elsevier Limited
© 2015, Elsevier Limited. All rights reserved.
First edition 1995 WB Saunders Ltd
Second edition 2005 Elsevier Ltd
Third edition 2015

Notices

Knowledge and best practice in this field are constantly changing. As new research and experience broaden our understanding, changes in research methods, professional practices, or medical treatment may become necessary.

Practitioners and researchers must always rely on their own experience and knowledge in evaluating and using any information, methods, compounds, or experiments described herein. In using such information or methods they should be mindful of their own safety and the safety of others, including parties for whom they have a professional responsibility.

With respect to any drug or pharmaceutical products identified, readers are advised to check the most current information provided (i) on procedures featured or (ii) by the manufacturer of each product to be administered, to verify the recommended dose or formula, the method and duration of administration, and contraindications. It is the responsibility of practitioners, relying on their own experience and knowledge of their patients, to make diagnoses, to determine dosages and the best treatment for each individual patient, and to take all appropriate safety precautions.

To the fullest extent of the law, neither the Publisher nor the authors, contributors, or editors, assume any liability for any injury and/or damage to persons or property as a matter of products liability, negligence or otherwise, or from any use or operation of any methods, products, instructions, or ideas contained in the material herein.

ISBN: 978-0-7020-4232-4

e-book ISBN: 978-0-7020-5031-2

Printed in China

Last digit is the print number: 9 8 7 6 5 4 3 2 1

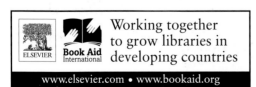

Working together
to grow libraries in
developing countries

ELSEVIER   Book Aid International

www.elsevier.com • www.bookaid.org

Contents

Preface

This is not a book of orthopaedic radiology. It is a book designed solely to assist with the accurate assessment of the plain radiographs obtained in the Emergency Department. Since the second edition was published in 2005 we have listened to the feedback from our numerous teaching courses and to those working in our Emergency Departments. Also, we recognise the plain film needs of present day radiologists in training. As a consequence we have placed a renewed emphasis on illustrating normal skeletal anatomy by utilising skilful and clarifying artworks. We have separated the common everyday injuries from those that occur much less frequently. First and foremost, we have adhered to our primary objective which is to assist all those who read Emergency Department radiographs and who ask the question… *"at first glance these images look normal to me—but how should I check them out in a logical and systematic manner?"*

The previous edition of the *Survival Guide* has proven to be helpful to Emergency Department doctors, Emergency Nurse Practitioners, Radiologists in training, Reporting Radiographers, and to General Practitioners working on their own in remote locations. We hope that this edition, with its improvements in content, in anatomical detail, in design and in layout, will once again assist all those who read, report, and depend upon accurate plain film interpretation in the Emergency Department.

Nigel Raby, Laurence Berman, Simon Morley, Gerald de Lacey
January 2014

Acknowledgements

We owe a prodigious amount of thanks to key individuals without whom this third edition would not have been completed. Claire Wanless created the new design and her editorial guidance has been masterly and absolutely invaluable. Philip Wilson produced the exquisite drawings that are a key part of each and every chapter. Jeremy Weldon, Consultant radiographer at Northwick Park Hospital helped us with the illustrative cases and he carried out the laboratory work on penetrating and swallowed foreign bodies. Dr Denis Remedios, Consultant radiologist at Northwick Park Hospital provided many original suggestions. Michael Houston, senior commissioning editor at Elsevier Ltd, prompted us to produce this third edition and facilitated and assisted us in our endeavours.

Our thanks are also due to a large and anonymous group, comprising doctors, radiographers, and radiologists in training who have attended our courses (www.radiology-courses.com and www.xraysurvivalguide.org), and through their constructive feedback have stimulated us to enhance numerous aspects, both large and small, in every chapter.

*"That is the essence of science:
ask an impertinent question and you are on the way to a pertinent answer."*

J. Bronowski, The Ascent of Man, 1973.

1 Key principles

Basic radiology

Describing injuries

Introduction

Patients with traumatic injuries can be placed into one of three major groups. The imaging approach will differ between these groups.

Polytrauma (in which one injury may be life threatening)

■ Imaging:

Strict local protocols and algorithms utilising early ultrasound (US) and/or multidetector computed tomography (CT). The use of plain film radiology in the Emergency Department (ED) is generally limited[1–4].

Multiple injuries (none of which is life threatening)

■ Imaging:

Plain film radiology is utilised in the ED.

Single injury (not life threatening)

■ Imaging:

Plain film radiology is the principal imaging investigation.

This book describes the assessment and interpretation of the plain radiographs that are customarily obtained in patients who have not sustained a life threatening injury.

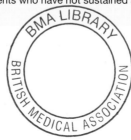

Key principles

Basic radiology

The radiographic image

The tissues that lie in the path of the X-ray beam absorb (ie attenuate) X-rays to differing degrees. These differences account for the radiographic image.

Attenuation of the X-ray beam

Tissue absorption		Effect on the radiograph
Least		
	Air or gas	Black image
	Fat	Dark grey image
	Soft tissue	Grey image
	Bone or calcium	White image
Most		

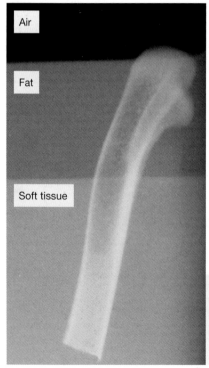

Air

Fat

Soft tissue

Radiograph of a chicken leg (bone) partially submerged in a layer of vegetable oil (fat) floating on water (soft tissue). Note the difference in the blackening of the X-ray film due to absorption by the different tissues.

Fracture lines: usually black, but sometimes white

When a fracture results in separation of bone fragments, the X-ray beam that passes through the gap is not absorbed by bone. This results in a black (ie lucent) line on the radiograph.

On the other hand, bone fragments may overlap or impact into each other. The resultant increased thickness of bone absorbs more of the X-ray beam and so results in a white (ie sclerotic or denser) area on the radiograph.

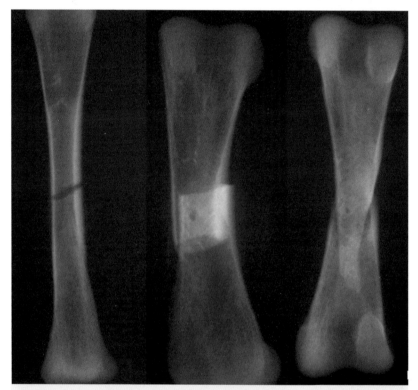

Three fractures. On the left the fragments are distracted and the fracture shows as a dark black line. In the centre the fragments overlap resulting in a dense region on the radiograph. On the right the fragments are impacted, also producing a dense region.

Fat pads and fluid levels

There are radiological soft tissue signs which can provide a clue that a fracture is likely. These include displacement of the elbow fat pads (see pp. 97 and 102), or the presence of a fat–fluid level at the knee joint (see pp. 248–249).

Key principles

The principle of two views

'One view only is one view too few'

Many fractures and dislocations are not detectable on a single view. Consequently, it is normal practice to obtain two standard projections, usually at right angles to each other. The example below shows two views of an injured finger.

At sites where fractures are known to be exceptionally difficult to detect (for example a suspected scaphoid fracture), it is routine practice to obtain more than two views.

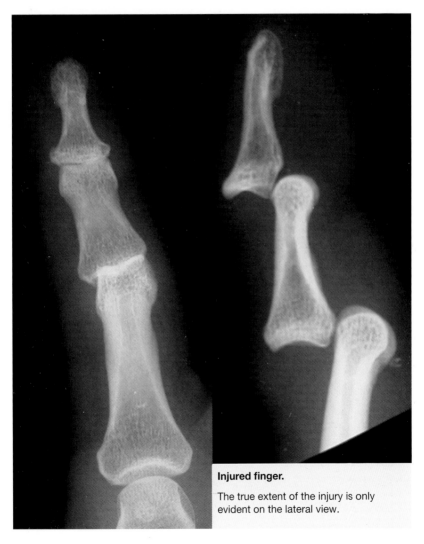

Injured finger.

The true extent of the injury is only evident on the lateral view.

Important information: patient position

Knowledge of the patient's position during radiography is essential. A radiograph obtained with the patient lying supine may produce a very different appearance when compared with the image acquired with the patient erect.

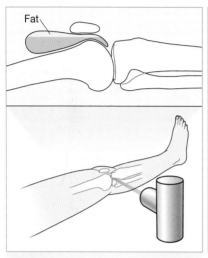

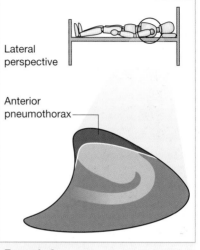

Lateral perspective

Anterior pneumothorax

Example 1.

Injured knee. Patient supine. A fat–fluid level in the suprapatellar bursa (p. 249) will only be seen when the radiograph is obtained with a horizontal X-ray beam. A vertical beam radiograph will not demonstrate the fat–fluid level.

Example 2.

A small pneumothorax will usually be detectable at the apex of the lung on an erect chest X-ray (CXR). On a supine CXR you need to look much lower down, ie around the heart, the diaphragm, and at the costophrenic angle[5].

Assessing the radiographs: discipline is essential

Missed injuries are common following trauma[6–9]. Detection of a fracture, and the components of a complex injury, depends on adherence to three cardinal rules:

- **Rule 1**. Always analyse both views.

- **Rule 2**. Develop a systematic step-by-step checking process for each radiograph even if a single abnormality is obvious. Two associated abnormalities often occur. The major danger: you can be seduced by the satisfaction of search phenomenon ("Yes—I have found the abnormality!"), and consequently a second important abnormality is overlooked.

- **Rule 3**. Check whether radiographs from the past exist. A change in appearance will often assist you in recognising an important abnormality. Similarly, an unchanged appearance may stop you from erroneously diagnosing a new injury or fracture[10].

Describing injuries

Fractures of the long bones

The radiographic appearance of a fracture needs to be described in a consistent style using accepted terminology. Imagine that you are describing a fracture of a long bone to the surgeon over the telephone[11–13]. These are the features the surgeon will want you to describe—simply and accurately:

- **Site.**

- **Closed or open.**

- **Fragments.**

- **Direction of the fracture.**

- **Articular surface involvement.**

- **Position of the two major fragments.**

- **Angulation.**

- **Rotational deformity.**

Site.

Specify which bone and which part of the bone. The shaft of a long bone is divided into thirds:

- Proximal.

- Middle.

- Distal.

Left: Fracture of distal third.

Right: Fracture at junction of proximal and middle thirds.

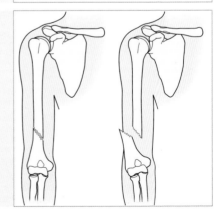

Closed or open.

- Closed: the fracture has not punctured the skin; no open wound (left).

- Open: the bone has pierced the skin (right). Also referred to as a compound fracture.

Fragments.

▪ Commreferenceition: more than two fragments (left).

▪ Impaction: one fragment is driven into the other (right).

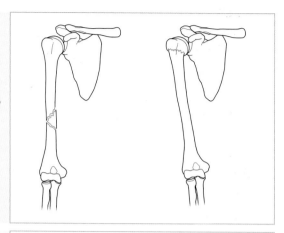

Direction of the fracture.

▪ Transverse: at right angles to the long axis of the bone (left).

▪ Oblique: at an angle of less than 90° to the long axis of the bone (middle).

▪ Spiral: curving and twisting along the bone (right).

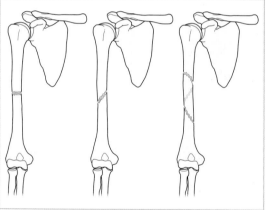

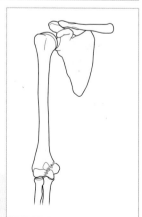

Articular surface involvement.

If a joint surface is involved the fracture is intra-articular.

Key principles

Position of the two major fragments.

Displaced or undisplaced.

Displacement is always described in relation to the distal fragment.

- Lateral displacement (left)

- No displacement (middle two images)

- Posterior displacement (right)

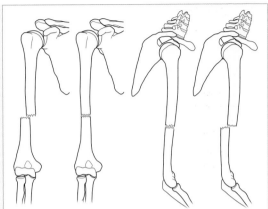

Angulation.

Describe[11,14] in relation to the distal fragment. Refer either to the direction in which the apex of the fracture points or to the direction of tilt of the distal fragment. Describing the direction of tilt may be easiest, as follows:

- Lateral tilt (left)

- Medial tilt (middle)

- Anterior tilt (right)

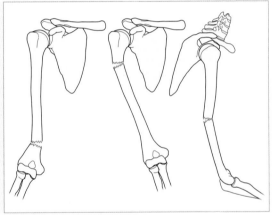

Rotational deformity.

A fragment has rotated on its long axis. Rotation may be external (left) or internal (right). Spontaneous correction is rare and surgery is usually required.

NB: Rotation of a fragment on its long axis is diagnosed most reliably by clinical examination. However, fragment rotation may be evident on the radiographs.

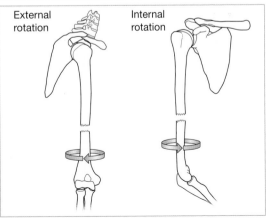

External rotation

Internal rotation

Dislocations

Precise use of language is important when describing subluxations and dislocations.

Subluxation

The joint surfaces are no longer congruous but the articular surface of one bone maintains some contact with the articular surface of the adjacent bone.

Example: inferior subluxation of the humeral head.

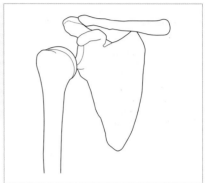

Dislocation

The articular surfaces at the joint have lost all contact with each other.

Example: inferior dislocation of the humeral head.

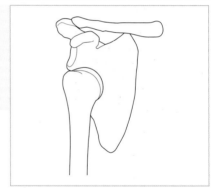

Normal joint

For reference.

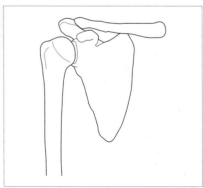

9

References

1. Pohlenz O, Bode PJ. The trauma emergency room: a concept for handling and imaging the polytrauma patient. Eur J Radiol 1996; 22: 2–6.
2. Hessmann MH, Hofmann A, Kreitner KF et al. The benefit of multislice CT in the Emergency Room management of polytraumatized patients. Acta Chir Belg 2006; 106: 500–507.
3. Kam CW, Lai CH, Lam SK et al. What are the ten new commandments in severe polytrauma management? World J Emerg Med 2010; 1: 85–92.
4. The Royal College of Radiologists. Standards of practice and guidance for trauma radiology in severely injured patients. London. The Royal College of Radiologists. 2011.
5. de Lacey G, Morley S, Berman L. The Chest X-Ray: A Survival Guide. Philadelphia, Saunders Elsevier, 2008. ISBN 978-0-7020-3046-8
6. Roberts CS. The missed injury in our big, flat, spiky world. Editorial. Injury 2008; 39: 1093–1094.
7. Guly HR. Diagnostic errors in an accident and emergency department. Emerg Med J 2001; 18: 263–269.
8. Pinto A, Brunese L. Spectrum of diagnostic errors in radiology. World J Radiol 2010; 28: 377–383.
9. Gatt ME, Spectre G, Paltiel O et al. Chest radiographs in the emergency department: is the radiologist really necessary? Postgrad Med J 2003; 79: 214–217.
10. Keats TE, Anderson MW. Atlas of normal Roentgen variants that may simulate disease, 9th ed. Elsevier Health Sciences, 2012.
11. Pitt MJ, Speer DP. Radiologic reporting of skeletal trauma. Radiol Clin North Am 1990; 28: 247–256.
12. Renner RR, Mauler GG, Ambrose JL. The radiologist, the orthopedist, the lawyer, and the fracture. Semin Roentgenol 1978; 13: 7–19.
13. Adam A, Dixon AK, Grainger RG, Allison DJ (eds): Grainger & Allison's Diagnostic Radiology. 5th ed. Churchill Livingstone/Elsevier, 2008.
14. Gaskin JSH, Pimple MK, Wharton R et al. How accurate and reliable are doctors in estimating fracture angulation? Injury 2007; 38: 160–162.

2 Particular paediatric points

Bones in children are different

Fracture sites

Sports injuries

Chest emergencies

Child abuse

Paediatric Points addressed in other chapters

Bones in children are different[1–4]

"A child is not a small adult..."

This truism is particularly important in relation to paediatric bone injuries[1]

Child versus adult

There are three major differences between a child's and an adult's skeleton[2–4].

1. Children have growth plates that:

   ❑ have the consistency of hard rubber and act, in part, as shock absorbers

   ❑ protect the joint surface from sustaining a comminuted fracture

   ❑ are weaker than the ligaments. Consequently the epiphysis will separate before a dislocation (ie ligamentous disruption) occurs.

2. Children have a thick periosteum that:

   ❑ is not only thick but very, very, strong

   ❑ acts as a hinge, which inhibits displacement when a fracture occurs.

3. Children's bones have an inherently different structure to adults' bones, being:

   ❑ less brittle

   ❑ flexible, elastic, and plastic, allowing an injured bone to bend or to buckle.

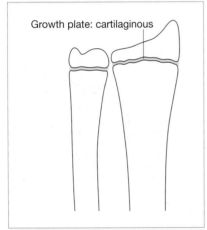

The growth plate (ie the physis) is a site of weakness.

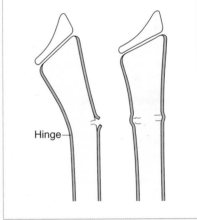

The very strong periosteum inhibits and impedes displacement at the site of the fracture.

The end of a long bone in a child

You need to be familiar with the normal radiographic appearance of the ends of the long bones in children. This will help you to detect the important injuries and will also protect you from labelling a normal developmental appearance as being abnormal.

A persistent lucent line is normal

A child's long bone grows in length initially by forming layers of cartilage and gradually converting that cartilage into bone. This layering process takes place at the end of the bone at the site of the physis (also called the epiphyseal plate or the growth plate). The physis is made of cartilage and lies between the epiphysis and the diaphysis. Cartilage is lucent on a radiograph. The cartilaginous physis remains as a radiographic lucency until the child reaches skeletal maturity and stops growing. At that time the lucent physis fuses to the metaphysis (and also to the epiphysis). When fusion occurs the linear lucency that was the physis disappears.

Parts of the skeleton are not missing

An epiphysis is a secondary centre of ossification at the end of a long bone. Each epiphysis is initially composed solely of cartilage. As a consequence it looks as though nothing is there (take a look at a new born baby's elbow region). Of course each of the epiphyses is present, but present as a radiolucent blob of cartilage. These invisible blobs enlarge slowly with age. Eventually they begin to ossify at their centres and become visible. Finally, these blobs of bone will fuse to the physis at maturity.

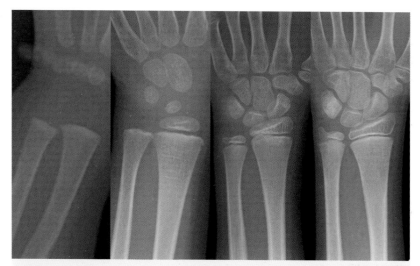

Normal wrist (left to right) in a young male at ages: 7 months; 5 years; 10 years; 14 years. Gradually the invisible epiphyses become ossified and consequently visible.

Fracture sites[1,3]

*"The key to accurate diagnosis is
a precisely accurate assessment of the radiographs."*[2]

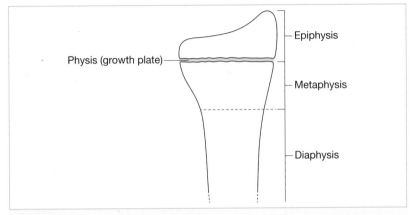

The anatomical regions in a long bone.

Epiphyseal–metaphyseal (Salter–Harris) fractures

The growth plate (the physis) is a very vulnerable structure. The joint capsule, the surrounding ligaments and the muscle tendons are all much stronger than the cartilaginous physis.

A shearing or avulsion force applied to a joint is most likely to result in an injury at the weakest point, ie a fracture through the growth plate.

Most growth plate injuries will heal well without any resultant deformity. However, in a few patients, failure to recognise a growth plate injury may result in suboptimal treatment with a risk of premature fusion resulting in limb shortening. If only a part of the growth plate is injured, unequal growth may lead to deformity and disability.

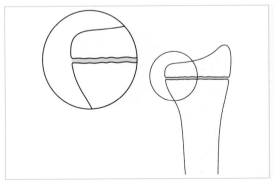

The cartilaginous growth plate (the physis) is a weak and vulnerable site in a long bone.

Injuries affecting the physis are common.

The Salter–Harris classification

This classification links the radiographic appearance of the fracture to the clinical importance of the fracture. A Salter–Harris type 1 injury has a good prognosis whereas a Salter–Harris type 5 injury has a poor prognosis.

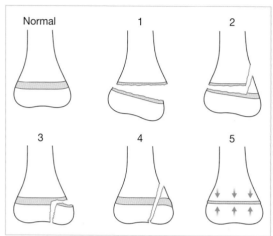

Salter–Harris fractures.

Type 1 is a fracture restricted to the growth plate.

Types 2–4 represent various patterns of fracture involving the growth plate and the adjacent metaphysis and/or epiphysis.

Type 5 is an impaction fracture of the entire growth plate.

Salter–Harris fractures

Type	Relative frequency	Prognosis for normal growth[4,5]	
		Upper limb	Lower limb
1	8%	Satisfactory	The likelihood of a growth complication is higher for all types of Salter–Harris injury as compared with the upper limb.
2	73%	Satisfactory	
3	6%	Satisfactory	
4	12%	Guarded	
5	1%	Poor	

How to remember the Salter–Harris (SH) classification

SH 1	= S	is **Separated** (a widened physis)
SH 2	= A	is **Above** the growth plate
SH 3	= L	is **beLow** the growth plate
SH 4	= T	is **Through** the growth plate
	= E	is for nothing!
SH 5	= R	has a **Rammed** together growth plate

Particular paediatric points

Salter–Harris fracture: five types

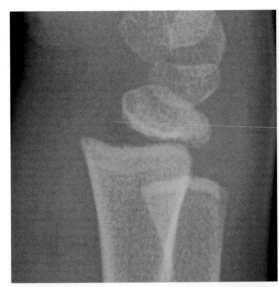

Type 1.

Fracture restricted to the growth plate. In this patient the epiphysis is displaced posteriorly.

Note: Many type 1 fractures do not show displacement of the epiphysis, making it impossible to detect the injury to the growth plate from the radiographs. Prognosis in these cases is invariably very good.

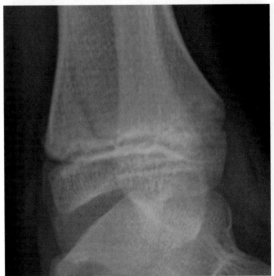

Type 2.

Fracture through the metaphysis that extends into the growth plate.

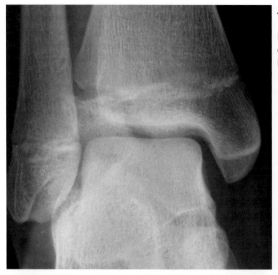

Type 3.

Fracture through the epiphysis that extends into the growth plate.

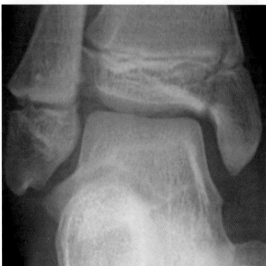

Type 4.

Fracture that involves the growth plate and the epiphysis and the metaphysis.

Type 4 runs the risk of premature fusion of part of the growth plate.

Type 5.

Impaction fracture of the entire growth plate. There is little or no malalignment and it is usually impossible to make the diagnosis on the initial radiographs. This is the most significant of the Salter–Harris injuries. The plate may fuse prematurely with consequent limb shortening. The diagnosis, and consequently optimal management, depends on a high degree of suspicion following clinical examination.

Metaphyseal–diaphyseal fractures

When a child's long bone is subjected to a longitudinal compression force (such as a fall on an outstretched hand), this can result in two common but different types of injury in the region of the metaphysis and proximal diaphysis.

▦ Torus fracture

▦ Greenstick fracture

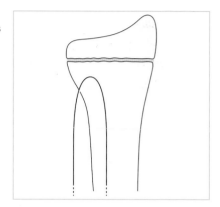

Torus fracture.

Results from a longitudinal compression force with little or no angulation. The axial loading is distributed evenly across the metaphysis (right). There are microfractures of the trabeculae at the injured site.

The commonest sites for a torus fracture are the distal radius and/or ulna.

The fracture is often subtle and appears as a ripple, a wave, an indent or a slight bump/bulge in the cortex. The bulge may be seen at both cortices or at one cortex only.

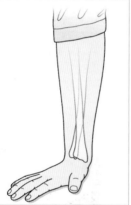

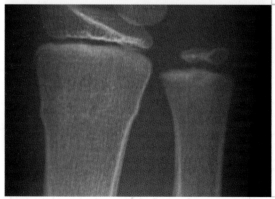

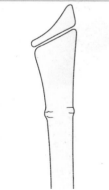

Fractures: some synonyms[3]

- Torus fracture = Buckle fracture
- Greenstick fracture = Angled Buckle fracture

The word "Torus" is derived from the latin word for a bulge.

Greenstick fracture.

A Greenstick fracture results from an angulation force.

There is a break in the cortex on one side of the bone. The opposite cortex remains intact. This occurs because of the very thick and elastic periosteum.

There is usually some angulation at the fracture site, although this can be slight and subtle.

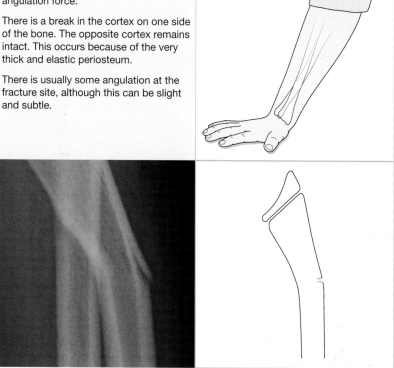

Particular paediatric points

Diaphyseal fractures[6,7]

A diaphyseal fracture: a break in the shaft of a long bone, well away from an epiphysis.

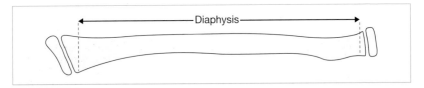
Diaphysis

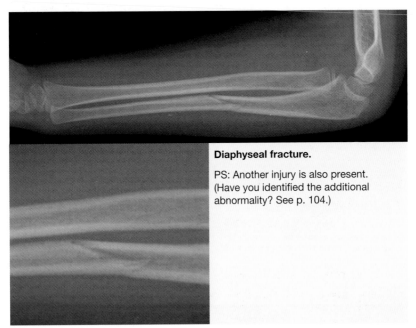

Diaphyseal fracture.

PS: Another injury is also present. (Have you identified the additional abnormality? See p. 104.)

Incomplete diaphyseal fracture —the plastic bowing fracture[1,7].

A child's bone may bend or bow with no obvious break in the cortex.

Traumatic bowing occurs as follows: a compression force extends along the longitudinal axis of the bone. The concave surface develops a series of microfractures causing the bone to bend. The compression force is insufficient to cause a transverse fracture.

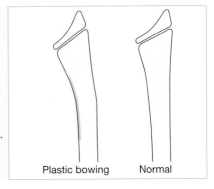

Plastic bowing   Normal

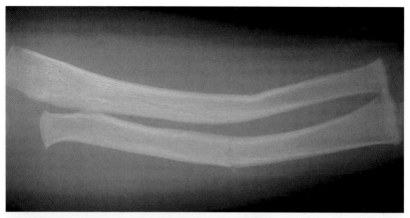

Plastic bowing fracture of the ulna.

There is an associated Greenstick fracture of the radius.

Plastic bowing fractures usually involve the radius or ulna but may affect other long bones including the femur, fibula, tibia, and occasionally the clavicle.

A plastic bowing fracture is sometimes known as a "bone bending fracture".

Diagnosing plastic bowing fractures.

Sometimes a bowing (or bending) injury can be difficult to diagnose with certainty because differences in radiographic positioning of the normal forearm bones can mimic a slightly bent bone. If you think that an injured bone is slightly bent then this justifies obtaining images of the opposite normal side. Comparison may make the bowing of the injured bone obvious.

A plastic bowing fracture may only be recognised in retrospect when subsequent radiographs show remodelling on the concave side of the bone.

Note: do not expect profuse periosteal new bone formation during healing following a plastic bowing fracture[6]. It is more common for remodelling alone to occur.

Particular paediatric points

Toddler's fracture[8-10]

The classic toddler's fracture involves the shaft of the tibia. Usually it occurs in a child aged 9 months to 3 years. The child falls with one leg fixed and a twisting injury occurs resulting in a spiral fracture of the tibia.

Invariably, the fracture is undisplaced and is frequently very difficult to visualise on the initial radiographs. Sometimes it will only be demonstrated on an additional oblique projection, or on a radionuclide study. If a repeat radiograph is obtained 10–14 days after the injury periosteal new bone will be present.

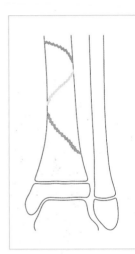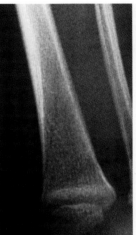

Toddler's fracture.

The undisplaced fracture spirals along the shaft of the distal tibia.

Clinical impact guideline: acute fractures in a limping toddler

The most common fracture is a spiral fracture of the shaft of the tibia —a "Toddler's fracture".

Other acute fractures do occur in limping toddlers. Fractures of the femur, cuboid, calcaneum, and distal fibula have all been described[8-13]. Different falling or stumbling mechanisms create particular forces that affect specific bones.

Because of the very similar history of a seemingly mild injury, and because all of these fractures can be radiographically very difficult to detect, it has been suggested that the collective term "Toddler's fractures" should be applied to this entire group of injuries[10]. This suggestion has gone unheeded.

The singular term "Toddler's fracture" persists, remains a specific term, and is applied solely to the classic spiral fracture of the tibia.

Clinical impact guideline: a limping toddler—what to do?

If a child refuses to weight-bear or is well but limping, then the possibility of a Toddler's fracture needs to be considered. If the tibia appears normal[8,13] on the digital images—including additional oblique views—then there are two possible courses of action:

- Scintigraphy will show whether a fracture is or is not present

  Or:

- Adopt an expectant approach. Toddler's fractures heal without any particular treatment. In a limping but otherwise well child who has sustained a Toddler's fracture, plain film radiography 10–14 days later will show evidence of the healing fracture (ie periosteal new bone formation).

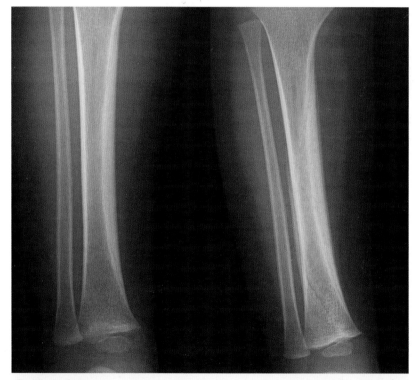

Toddler's fracture.

The original radiograph (left) obtained when the child first started to limp was passed as normal. Ten days later the radiograph (right) shows the fracture as well as extensive periosteal new bone extending along the full length of the tibia.

Particular paediatric points

Sports injuries[14–17]

Sports injuries affecting young children and adolescents are common. Some of these patients will attend the Emergency Department complaining of acute or chronic pain.

Acute Injuries

Acute fractures follow the same patterns as those that occur as a result of accidental trauma in the playground or elsewhere. Salter–Harris growth plate fractures, Torus and Greenstick fractures, and plastic bowing fractures are described on pp. 14–21.

Chronic injuries

A chronic sports injury may cause diagnostic difficulty to the unwary. Three skeletal injuries occur: stress fractures, avulsion fractures, and osteochondral injuries.

Stress fractures[15–20]

Most stress fractures occur in the lower limbs as a consequence of weight bearing stresses in runners and footballers. Other activities can affect the ribs and upper limbs. The appearances of stress fractures on plain radiographs do vary.

Scintigraphy will detect a stress fracture when the plain radiographs appear normal.

MRI is the most sensitive test for identifying fractures in their very earliest stages[19]. If there is clinical suspicion of a stress fracture and the plain radiographs appear normal then MRI is the imaging test of choice; it will provide the maximum detail in relation to the fracture.

Stress fractures[14,15,17,18]

Bone	Site	Recognised activities
Pelvis	Pubic ramus	Distance runners, gymnasts
Femur	Shaft/neck	Dancers
Tibia	Proximal third or junction of mid & dist thirds	Runners, footballers, dancers
Fibula	Distal third	Runners, footballers
Navicular	Centre	Runners, jumpers, footballers
Calcaneum		Jumpers
Metatarsals	Shafts	Dancers, runners, footballers
Sesamoids		Runners
Wrist	Growth plate	Gymnasts
Vertebrae L4 or L5	Pars interarticularis	Dancers, fast bowlers, gymnasts, tennis players, USA football linemen
Ribs	First rib	Throwers

Note: Stress fractures are not limited to these sites nor these activities only.

Radiographic appearances of stress fractures

Early	Normal
2-4 weeks	Variable findings:
	▪ Hairline fracture
	▪ Vague cortical lucency
	▪ Periosteal new bone formation
Later	Callus and endosteal reaction

If not recognised or treated, a stress fractures will sometimes progress to a complete and displaced fracture.

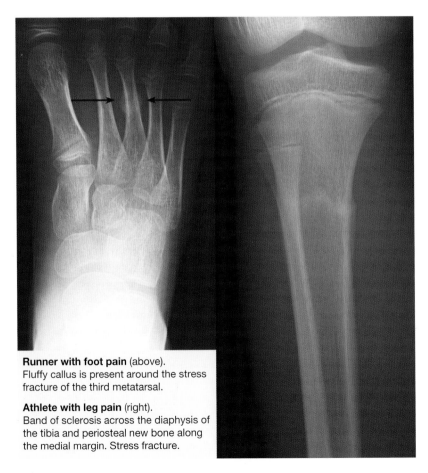

Runner with foot pain (above).
Fluffy callus is present around the stress fracture of the third metatarsal.

Athlete with leg pain (right).
Band of sclerosis across the diaphysis of the tibia and periosteal new bone along the medial margin. Stress fracture.

Particular paediatric points

Avulsion injuries[15,16,21,22]

Apophyseal fractures occur almost exclusively in athletic children and adolescents[21,22]. Hurdling, sprinting, soccer, and tennis are the principal at-risk activities.

An apophysis is a secondary ossification centre that is not related to a joint surface. Consequently, an apophyseal fracture is a growth plate injury and is analogous to a Salter–Harris type 1 fracture. Apophyses are often the sites of tendonous insertions and avulsion occurs as a result of a violent or repetitive muscle pull. The most common avulsion sites are:

- Ischial tuberosity

- Anterior inferior iliac spine (AIIS)

- Anterior superior iliac spine (ASIS)

- Humerus: medial epicondyle. (Incidentally this is not an apophysis. It is an epiphysis.) Nevertheless, avulsion is fairly common at the elbow. It represents the so-called "little leaguer's elbow" because throwing sports can cause the medial epicondyle to be pulled off. These activities include baseball pitching.

For additional detail about avulsion injuries at particular sites see:

- Pelvis—p. 224.

- Elbow—p. 105.

- Midfoot and forefoot—p. 298.

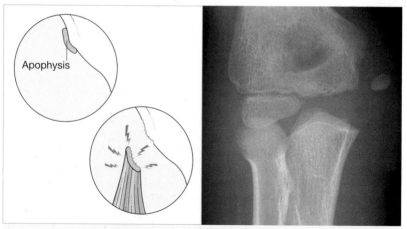

Apophysis

An apophysis can be avulsed from the parent bone by repetitive vigorous muscle contraction (left). Similarly, the medial epicondyle secondary centre can be detached (right) during throwing sports. Also, this avulsion is often consequent when a violent valgus stress is sustained during a fall onto an outstretched hand.

Pelvic avulsion injuries are common. Radiographic appearances...

Acute:

- An ossified apophyseal fragment is detached and visible

Chronic:

- Variable appearances:
  - Apophyseal irregularity
  - Sclerotic and fragmented apophysis
  - Exuberant callus
  - Calcification in a surrounding haematoma
- The Golden Rule:
  - Always compare the painful side with the opposite and normal side

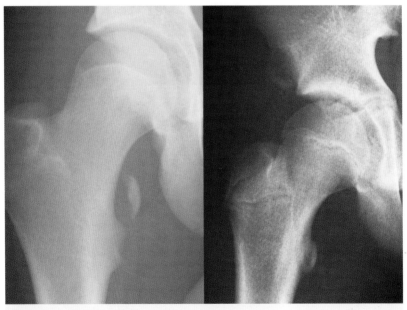

Two young athletes with hip pain.

Avulsed femoral apophysis (left). Avulsed right AIIS (right).

Particular paediatric points

Chondral & osteochondral injuries[14,15]

Repetitive trauma with impaction of one cartilage covered bone on another can cause fissuring within the underlying bone. A defect may result and a lucency within the affected bone can become visible on the radiograph. The lesion is termed osteochondritis dissecans (OCD). Sometimes a bone fragment becomes loose and may be seen within the joint. The sites most commonly affected are the:

- lateral aspect of the medial femoral condyle
- medial and lateral margins of the talus
- capitellum of the distal humerus.

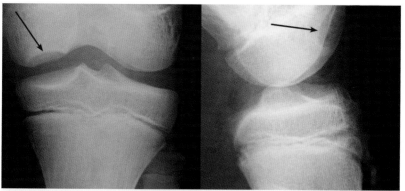

OCD in the medial condyle of the femur (arrows). The position is typical for this lesion.

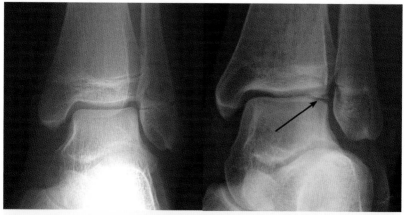

Normal smooth cortex of the dome of the talus (left).

Osteochondral fracture of the lateral aspect of the talar dome (right).

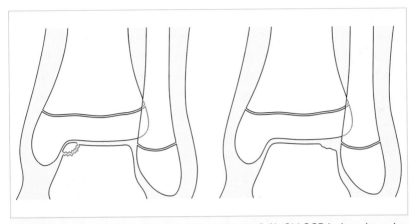

Acute or recently acquired osteochondritis dissecans (left). Old OCD lesion, shown by an irregular defect in the articular surface of the talus (right).

The talar dome is a vulnerable site.

Summary: osteochondritis dissecans

Description. An area of bone at a joint surface becomes separated from the rest of the bone surrounding it. The bone fragment, with its cartilage cap, becomes loose. It represents a fragment lying within a crater. The fragment may break off and become completely free within the joint.

Aetiology. Several different possibilities have been suggested including a genetic disposition as the primary cause. The blood supply to the affected bone fragment is damaged. There is little doubt that repetitive trauma with impaction of one bone on another is the major cause in many instances[14,15].

Common sites. Medial condyle of the distal femur; lateral or medial aspects of the dome of the tarsal talus; the capitellum of the distal humerus.

Symptoms. Joint pain. Sometimes a detached fragment lying loose within the joint will cause the joint to lock.

Additional imaging. MRI will determine whether the articular cartilage overlying the bone fragment is intact. This information can influence the precise choice of management of a particular lesion.

Chest emergencies[23-26]

Children attend the Emergency Department with upper and lower airway problems including coughing, chest trauma, wheezing, and pneumonia. The plain film radiology of these problems is addressed in *The Chest X-Ray: A Survival Guide*[24].

For swallowed foreign bodies, see pp. 349–362.

Inhaled foreign body

Infants and toddlers are at risk of foreign body aspiration, frequently unwitnessed. The most commonly inhaled foreign body is food, often a peanut[23,25,27-30]. A history of choking is usually obtained. Common clinical signs include coughing, stridor, wheezing and sternal retraction. Rapid recognition and treatment are essential.

Radiography

If the child is able to cooperate then a frontal chest X-ray (CXR) should be obtained following a rapid forced expiration. Air trapping on the affected side (due to obstruction of the airway) is then more obvious.

Fluoroscopy is an excellent way of observing whether there is unilateral air trapping.

Possible findings on the CXR:

- Obstructive atelectasis—areas of collapse/consolidation.

- Obstructive emphysema—a unilateral hypertransradiant lung, due to air trapping. The affected lung appears blacker and larger than the opposite normal side.

- Normal appearances. This is not necessarily reassuring. If the clinical suspicion remains that a foreign body has been inhaled then an emergency MRI[28] or bronchoscopy is essential.

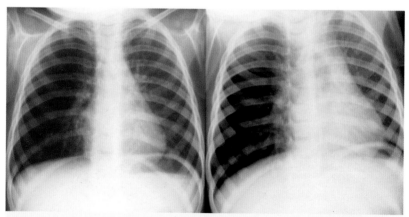

An inhaled peanut in the right main bronchus. Inspiration film (left): the right lung is hypertransradiant (ie blacker) compared with the left. Following rapid expiration (right), air trapping on the right is now obvious. Mediastinal displacement to the left is evident. Note: food (including peanuts) will not be visible on a radiograph.

Child abuse: skeletal injuries[31–34]

The possibility of non-accidental injury (NAI) must be considered in all injured children presenting to the Emergency Department. No socioeconomic group or race is exempt.

■ 50% of cases of NAI occur before the age of 1 year.

■ 80% of cases occur before the age of 2 years.

Normal radiographs do not exclude the diagnosis. In 50% of proven cases of NAI the radiographs are normal. Nevertheless, fractures are the second most common finding in child abuse; second, after cutaneous abnormalities such as bruises and contusions.

Clinical and radiological involvement in suspected NAI

Usual requirements/practice:

■ Early involvement of the designated paediatric team.

■ The paediatric team takes responsibility for instigating and organising a skeletal survey when they deem this to be indicated.

■ Specialist paediatric radiologists review and report on all of the radiographs obtained.

■ All radiographs are double-read by two paediatric radiologists.

Under- and over-diagnosis of NAI[31,34]

Failure to diagnose a particular injury as being suggestive of abuse in a child attending the Emergency Department can have devastating consequences. Similarly, an over-diagnosis of NAI can be highly detrimental for the child and for those who are looking after the child. A particular area of difficulty is the evaluation of an infant's or toddler's skull radiographs because of the skull sutures (see pp. 36–45).

Radiological pitfalls in the diagnosis of NAI in the Emergency Department

1. Failure to consider the possibility of child abuse.

2. Ignorance of the particular or specific radiological features (ie appearance or position) that should raise the suspicion of NAI.

3. Normal skeletal variants misinterpreted as evidence of NAI. These include accessory skull sutures, physiological periosteal reaction, and normal metaphyseal variants[35].

4. Suboptimal imaging.

5. Other pathological processes, such as osteogenesis imperfecta, osteomyelitis and scurvy may simulate some of the skeletal features of NAI.

Radiographic features suggestive of NAI[31,32,34]

Subperiosteal new bone formation (right). Periosteal reactions may result from subperiosteal bleeding due to punching, shaking or squeezing. Periosteal reaction and callus formation can occur within a few days of trauma, but will not be present on the actual day of the injury. If new bone is present then some days or weeks have elapsed since the injury.

More than one fracture (not shown). Particularly suspicious if the stages of evolution of the fractures appear to be different, since this indicates that the injuries have occurred at different times. For example one fracture may show some faint periosteal new bone, whereas another may demonstrate mature callus.

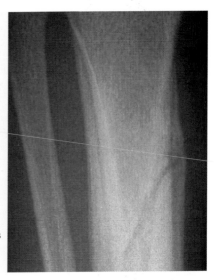

Radiographic features highly suggestive of NAI[31,32,34]

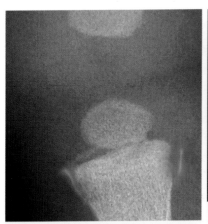

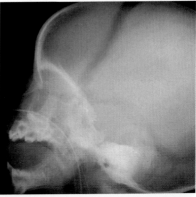

A small fracture at the corner of a metaphysis of a long bone.

This is known as a corner fracture.

Skull fractures that are wide (as in this child), complex and involving both sides of the skull, or involving both the occiput and the vertex.

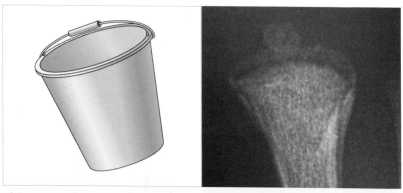

A transverse fracture of the distal metaphysis of a long bone.

This has been likened to a bucket handle, hence the term "bucket handle fracture".

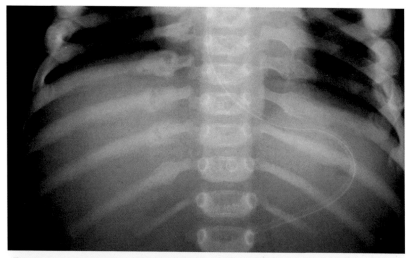

Fractures involving the posterior aspects of the ribs close to the spine.

These occur when a child is held by the chest and shaken or squeezed.

- Rib fractures in children under the age of 2 years are usually due to NAI.

- Rib fractures often result from very violent shaking episodes—these have a recognised association with brain injury.

Fractures of the pelvis, sternum, and the vertebral transverse processes.

These are rarely caused by an accidental injury.

References

1. Kirks DR, Griscom NT (eds). Practical pediatric imaging: diagnostic radiology of infants and children. 3rd ed. Lippincott Williams & Wilkins, 1998.
2. Conrad EU, Rang MC. Fractures and sprains. Ped Clin North Am 1986; 33: 1523–1540.
3. Swischuk LE. Subtle fractures in kids: how not to miss them. Applied Radiology 2002; 31: 15–19.
4. Kao SCS, Smith WL. Skeletal injuries in the pediatric patient. Radiol Clin North Am 1997; 35: 727–746.
5. Mizuta T, Benson WM, Foster BK et al. Statistical analysis of the incidence of physeal injuries. J Pediatr Orthop 1987; 7: 518–523.
6. Crowe JE, Swischuk LE. Acute bowing fractures of the forearm in children: a frequently missed injury. AJR 1977; 128: 981–984.
7. Attia MW, Glasstetter DS. Plastic bowing type fracture of the forearm in two children. Pediatr Emerg Care 1997; 13: 392–393.
8. Fahr MJ, James LP, Beck JR et al. Digital radiography in the diagnosis of Toddler's fracture. South Med J 2003; 96: 234–239.
9. Swischuk LE, John SD, Tschoepe EJ. Upper tibial hyperextension fractures in infants: another occult toddler's fracture. Pediat Radiol 1999; 29: 6–9.
10. John SD, Moorthy CS, Swischuk LE. Expanding the concept of the toddler's fracture. Radiographics 1997; 17: 367–376.
11. Blumberg K, Patterson RJ. The toddler's cuboid fracture. Radiology 1991; 179: 93–94.
12. Laliotis N, Pennie BH, Carty H et al. Toddler's fracture of the calcaneum. Injury 1993; 24: 169–170.
13. Donnelly LF. Toddler's fracture of the fibula. Am J Roentgenol 2000; 175: 922.
14. Long G. Imaging of paediatric sports injuries. RAD Magazine 1999; 26: 23–24.
15. Carty H. Sports injuries in children—a radiological viewpoint. Arch Dis Child 1994; 70: 457–460.
16. Anderson SJ. Lower extremity injuries in youth sports. Pediatr Clin North Am 2002; 49: 627–641.
17. Heyworth BE, Green DW. Lower extremity stress fractures in pediatric and adolescent athletes. Curr Opin Pediatr 2008; 20: 58–61.
18. Daffner RH, Pavlov H. Stress Fractures: Current Concepts. Am J Roentgenol 1992; 159: 245–252.
19. Daffner RH. MRI of occult and stress fractures. Applied Radiology 2003; 32: 40–49.
20. Connolly SA, Connolly LP, Jaramillo D. Imaging of sports injuries in children and adolescents. Radiol Clin North Am 2001; 39: 773–90.
21. Sundar M, Carty H. Avulsion fractures of the pelvis in children: a report of 32 fractures and their outcome. Skeletal Radiol 1994; 23: 85–90.
22. El-Khoury GY, Daniel WW, Kathol MH. Acute and chronic avulsive injuries. Radiol Clin North Am 1997; 35: 747–766.
23. Swischuk LE, John SD. Emergency pediatric chest radiology. Emerg Rad 1999; 6: 160–169.
24. de Lacey G, Morley S, Berman L. The Chest X-Ray: A Survival Guide. Philadelphia, Saunders Elsevier. 2008.
25. Chapman T, Sandstrom CK, Parnell SE. Pediatric emergencies of the upper and lower airway. Applied Radiology April 2012.
26. Carty H. Emergency Pediatric Radiology. Springer-Verlag, 2002.
27. Baharloo F, Veyckemans F, Francis C et al. Tracheobronchial foreign bodies: presentation and management in children and adults. Chest 1999; 115: 1357–1362.
28. Imaizumi H, Kaneko M, Nara S et al. Definitive diagnosis and location of peanuts in the airways using magnetic resonance imaging techniques. Ann Emerg Med 1994; 23: 1379–1382.
29. Sersar SI, Rizk WH, Bilal M et al. Inhaled Foreign Bodies: Presentation, Management and value of History and Plain Chest Radiography in Delayed Presentation. Otolaryngology—Head and Neck Surgery 2006; 134: 92–99.
30. Zaupa P, Saxena AK, Barounig A et al. Management Strategies in Foreign-Body Aspiration. Indian J Pediatr 2009; 76: 157–161.
31. Offiah A, van Rijn RR, Perez-Rossello JM et al. Skeletal Imaging of child abuse (non-accidental injury). Pediatr Radiol 2009; 39: 461–470.
32. Ebrahim N. Patterns and mechanisms of injury in non-accidental injury in children (NAI). SA Fam Pract 2008; 50: 5–13.
33. Kemp AM, Butler A, Morris S et al. Which radiological investigations should be performed to identify fractures in suspected child abuse? Clin Rad 2006; 61: 723–736.
34. Carty H, Pierce A. Non-accidental injury: a retrospective analysis of a large cohort. Eur Radiol 2002; 12: 2919–2925.
35. Kleinman PK. Diagnostic imaging in infant abuse. AJR 1990; 155: 703–712.

3 Paediatric skull —suspected NAI

Normal anatomy

Analysis: suture recognition

A skull X-ray (SXR) continues to have an important role when there is suspicion of non-accidental injury (NAI) in an infant or a toddler[1-3]. The primary indication for a SXR in these patients is forensic[3].

Be careful:

■ Accessory sutures are common.

■ Calling an accessory suture a fracture may lead to an incorrect suggestion of NAI.

■ Dismissing a fracture as an accessory suture can have serious clinical consequences.

■ To avoid mistakes:

❏ Be aware of the positions of the common accessory sutures.

❏ Assess and interpret an infant's or toddler's radiographs in a systematic step-by-step manner.

The standard radiographs

■ **Lateral.**

■ **AP frontal view.**

■ **Towne's view.**

The precise SXR views to be obtained will be specified by the local protocol for NAI assessment in infants and toddlers[3].

Abbreviations: the sutures

C, coronal;
In, innominate;
L, lambdoid;
M, mendosal;
Met, metopic;
O, occipitomastoid;
P1 and P2, accessory parietal;
Sa, sagittal;
Sq, squamosal.

NAI, non-accidental injury.

Normal anatomy

Infants and toddlers—normal accessory sutures

Evaluating the SXR in an infant or toddler presents unique problems. Diagnostic confusion between sutures and fractures may have serious consequences. A basic understanding of the locations and variable appearances of these sutures will help to reduce the likelihood of misdiagnosis[4-8].

A basic classification of skull sutures in infants and toddlers

Grouping	Notes	Sutures
The normal sutures	Visible on the SXR in all infants and toddlers – persisting in all adults	Sagittal, coronal, lambdoid, squamosal, and smaller sutures around the mastoid
A normal developmental suture	Visible on the SXR in all infants and many toddlers – but not in adults	Innominate
The most common accessory sutures	Visible on the SXR in some infants and toddlers – occasionally persisting to adulthood	Metopic, accessory parietal, mendosal

Normal accessory sutures and the radiographs on which they are seen

Suture	Most commonly seen on	Notes
Metopic suture	Frontal ℘ ℘ Towne's ℘	The commonest accessory suture. It is also the one that most commonly persists in older children, and even in a few adults.
Accessory parietal suture	Towne's ℘ ℘ Frontal ℘ Lateral ℘	May be complete or incomplete. Occurs in vertical, horizontal or oblique orientations. Most commonly vertical.
Mendosal suture	Lateral ℘ ℘ Towne's ℘	Extends posteriorly from the lambdoid suture on the lateral view. Passes medially on Towne's view.
Innominate suture	Lateral ℘ ℘	Sometimes classified as an accessory suture but best regarded as a normal developmental suture because it is always present in infants. As the child matures this suture disappears.

The lateral SXR

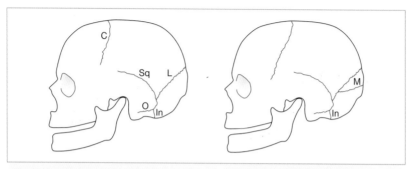

The normal sutures. L = lambdoid suture; C = coronal suture; M = mendosal;
O = occipitomastoid suture; Sq = squamosal suture; In = innominate suture

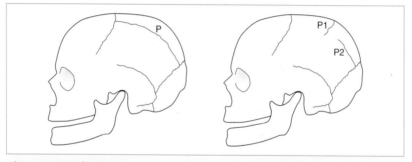

Accessory parietal sutures. Can appear in various positions (P).

Accessory parietal sutures vary in position. This drawing does not correspond to any radiographic projection. It shows the general positions and direction of the more common incomplete accessory parietal sutures (P1 and P2) when looking down from above the cranium.

L = lambdoid suture;

C = coronal suture;

Sa = sagittal suture;

P = accessory parietal sutures.

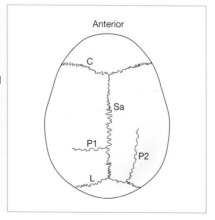

The AP frontal SXR

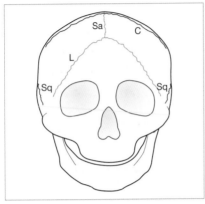

Normal sutures on the frontal view.

L = lambdoid suture;

C = coronal suture;

Sa = sagittal suture;

Sq = squamosal suture.

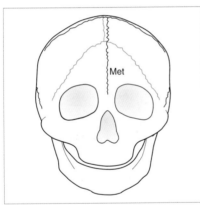

Accessory suture—the metopic.

This suture divides the frontal bone into two halves.

Met = metopic suture.

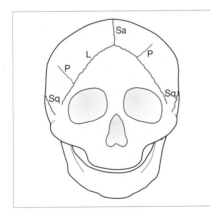

Accessory parietal sutures.

The drawing shows possible positions/sites of accessory parietal sutures.

L = lambdoid suture;

Sa = sagittal suture;

Sq = squamosal suture;

P = accessory parietal suture.

The Towne's SXR

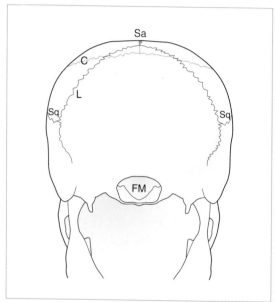

Normal sutures on the Towne's view.

L = lambdoid suture;

C = coronal suture;

Sa = sagittal suture;

Sq = squamosal suture;

FM = foramen magnum.

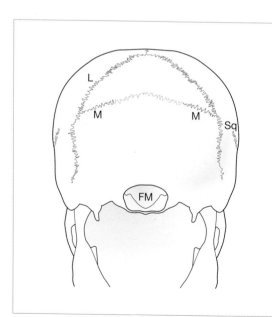

Accessory suture —the mendosal.

This accessory suture is situated in the occipital bone. Very occasionally it is whole (ie complete). More often it is incomplete. Very often it is incomplete and on one side of the bone only.

M = mendosal suture;

L = lambdoid suture;

Sq = squamosal suture;

FM = foramen magnum.

Analysis: suture recognition

The principal question: is it a suture or a fracture?[4-8]

When assessing suspected non-accidental injury (NAI) in young children, be very careful not to rush too swiftly to judgement. Observing an abnormality is important. An informed approach is then required when assigning a particular significance to the abnormality[9-12].

Be aware...

- Wide sutures are normal in neonates.

- Accessory sutures are common and are a part of normal development. An awareness of the positions and appearances of the common accessory sutures will help to reduce errors of interpretation.

- The age at which an accessory suture closes is variable. Accessory sutures are present in some older children. Very occasionally they persist into adulthood.

- Radiography in a wriggling infant can be very difficult. The Towne's view (injury to occiput) or the AP frontal view (injury elsewhere) is frequently a technical compromise. The head is often slightly rotated.

Assessing the radiographs

1. Trace every line seen on the two standard radiographs.
   For each line ask yourself: is this a suture?

2. Whenever a lucent line is detected it is essential to assess the two radiographs together. They form a complementary pair.

3. Always correlate the findings with the clinical history and the physical examination.

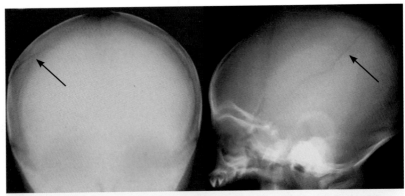

The importance of evaluating the two SXR views as a pair. On the frontal SXR (left) the lucent line (arrow) could be interpreted as an accessory suture. The lateral view (right) shows that the line (arrow) is much more extensive and continues through to the temporal bone. This is a fracture.

Suture recognition on the Towne's view

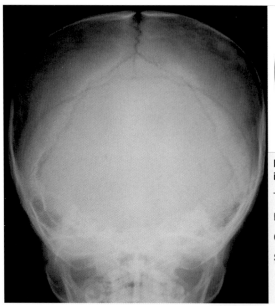

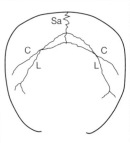

Normal sutures present in all children.

Towne's view.

L = lambdoid suture;

C = coronal suture;

Sa = sagittal suture.

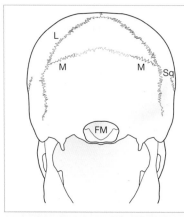

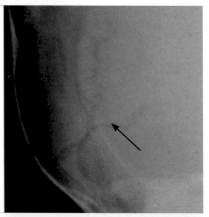

Mendosal suture. A mendosal suture (arrow) can be present on both sides. It may be complete or incomplete. Most commonly it is incomplete. M = mendosal suture; L = lambdoid suture; Sq = squamosal suture; FM = foramen magnum.

Suture recognition on the lateral view

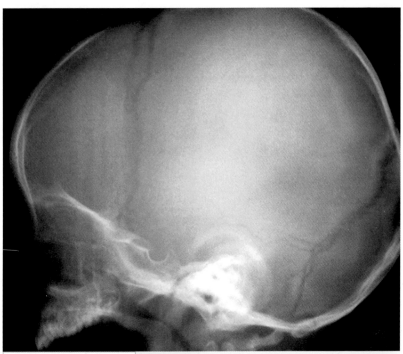

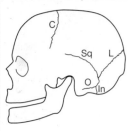

Lateral view.

L = lambdoid suture;
C = coronal suture;
O = occipitomastoid suture;
Sq = squamosal suture;
In = innominate suture.

The sagittal and metopic sutures are not seen on the lateral view because they lie in the midline (ie parallel to the plane of the radiograph).

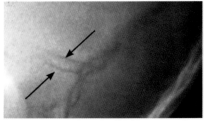

Squamosal suture. Extends anteriorly, separating the parietal bone from the temporal bone. The usual appearance is of a pair of lines (arrows) on the lateral projection (ie the left squamosal suture and the right squamosal suture). Invariably, the squamosal suture fades away as it passes anteriorly.

Lambdoid suture. As it nears the base of the skull (in the region of the mastoid bone) the suture appears to be complex. This seemingly tangled appearance is mainly caused by overlapping of the normal occipitomastoid sutures on the right and left sides. Don't worry about this. Arising from the lambdoid suture there will be:

- a normal suture,
  the **squamosal suture**.

- a *normal developmental suture*,
  the **innominate suture**.

- sometimes, an *accessory suture*,
  the **mendosal suture**.

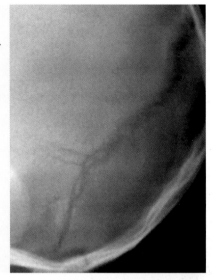

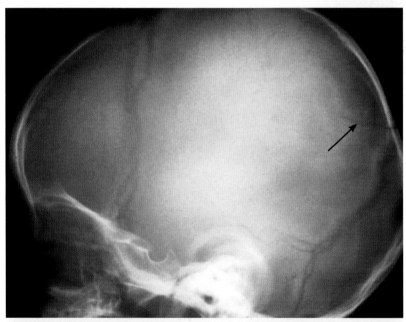

Accessory parietal sutures (also known as intraparietal sutures).

These are often best seen (arrow) on this view.

Suture recognition on the AP view

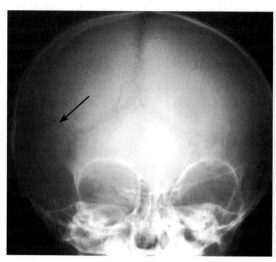

The sagittal and lambdoid sutures are well shown. In addition an accessory parietal suture (arrow) is also present.

The lambdoid suture meets the sagittal suture in the midline.

On the frontal radiograph the sagittal suture appears foreshortened.

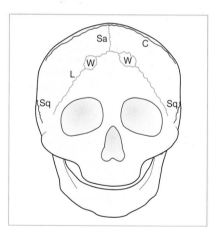

Normal sutures on the frontal view.

This diagram also shows wormian bones contained within the lambdoid sutures.

L = lambdoid suture;

C = coronal suture;

Sa = sagittal suture;

Sq = squamosal suture;

W = wormian bone.

Wormian bones.

It is not uncommon to see one (or several) wormian bones (W) on the AP projection, and occasionally also on other projections. This is a normal finding. A wormian bone is a small area of the skull (sometimes as large as 1–2 cm in diameter) within a suture. The bone is completely surrounded by the lucent suture.

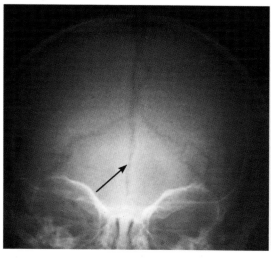

Metopic suture.

Where it meets the coronal suture, the sagittal suture should stop. If it continues below this point then the patient has a metopic suture. This accessory suture divides the frontal bone into two halves. The metopic suture (arrow) is the commonest accessory suture in children. Sometimes it persists into adulthood. Note the wormian bone in the sagittal suture and another in the left lambdoid suture.

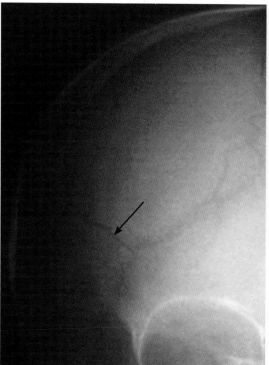

Accessory parietal suture.

Accessory parietal sutures are not exceptional. Of all the accessory sutures these are the ones that cause the most confusion.

Accessory parietal sutures may be complete or incomplete. They may be visualised on the frontal (arrow) and/or the lateral projections.

References

1. Head injury: Triage, assessment, investigation and early management of head injury in infants, children and adults. NICE Clinical guideline 56, 2007. http://www.nice.org.uk/nicemedia/pdf/CG56NICEGuideline.pdf
2. Reed MJ, Browning JG, Wilkinson AG, Beattie T. Can we abolish skull Xrays for head injury? Arch Dis Child 2005; 90: 859–864.
3. Jaspan T, Griffiths PD, McConachie NS, Punt JA. Neuroimaging for Non-Accidental Head Injury in Childhood: A Proposed Protocol. Clin Rad 2003; 58: 44–53.
4. Allen WE, Kier EL, Rothman SL. Pitfalls in the evaluation of skull trauma. A review. Radiol Clin North Am 1973; 11: 479–503.
5. Shapiro R. Anomalous parietal sutures and the bipartite parietal bone. AJR 1972; 115: 569–577.
6. Matsumura G, Uchiumi T, Kida K et al. Developmental studies on the interparietal part of the human occipital squama. J Anat 1993; 182: 197–204.
7. Billmire ME, Myers PA. Serious head injury in infants: accident or abuse? Pediatrics 1985; 75: 340–342.
8. Merten DF, Osborne DRS, Radkowski MA, Leonidas JC. Craniocerebral trauma in the child abuse syndrome: radiological observations. Pediatr Radiol 1984; 14: 272–277.
9. Lonergan GJ, Baker AM, Morey MK, Boos SC. Child abuse: Radiologic – pathologic correlation. Radiographics 2003; 23: 811–845.
10. Loder RT, Bookout C. Fracture patterns in battered children. J Orthop Trauma 1991; 5: 428–433.
11. King J, Diefendorf D, Apthorp J et al. Analysis of 429 fractures in 189 battered children. J Pediatr Orthop 1988; 8: 585–589.
12. Rao P, Carty H. Non-accidental injury: review of the radiology. Clin Radiol 1999; 54: 11–24.

4

Adult skull

Following a head injury the imaging examination of choice is CT[1-9].

Plain film skull radiography (SXR) has in the main been abandoned[6] or its use radically reduced as a first line imaging test both in children and in adults[1-4].

A SXR is now limited to:

- where national or local guidelines indicate a role within a patient management algorithm;

- locations where imaging resources are limited and CT is not available.

If a SXR is obtained there are just three abnormal features to look for: linear fractures, depressed fractures, and a fluid level in the sphenoid sinus.

The standard radiographs

Radiographs comprising a standard SXR series:

- A **Lateral** obtained with a horizontal X-ray beam, and one additional view depending on the site of injury.

  - Trauma to the occipital bone = **Towne's view**.

  - Any other injury = **PA frontal view**.

Abbreviations

CT, computed tomography; PA, posterior-anterior view; SXR, skull X-ray.

Following an apparently mild head injury requests for skull radiography (SXR) will occur very infrequently[1-9]. Compelling evidence that CT should be the examination of choice was initially based on a meta-analysis of 20 head injury surveys[7]. SXR series may still be requested, perhaps in remote locations where imaging facilities are limited.

Anatomy

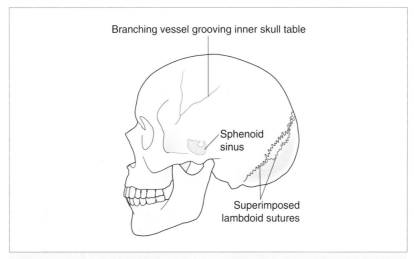

Normal features on a lateral SXR.

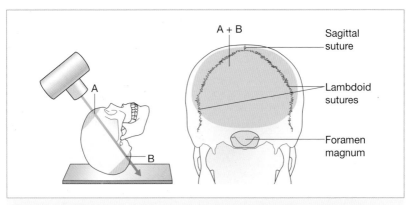

Towne's view. This radiograph is obtained primarily to show the occipital bone. Note that the frontal and occipital bones are superimposed on the image. A fracture through the frontal bone may therefore also be visualised on this radiograph.

Analysis: false positive diagnoses

Most difficulties with interpretation arise because a normal appearance can be mistaken for an abnormality. These false positive diagnoses can be reduced by being familiar with the following.

- The normal sutures and accessory sutures (pp. 36–39). Specifically, the position and appearance of:
  - the three large sutures: the lambdoid, coronal and sagittal;
  - the other smaller sutures around the mastoid bones.
- The metopic suture (p. 38). The most common accessory suture persisting in some adults.
- Vascular impressions. Specifically:
  - the sites of the most common vessel grooves/markings;
  - the radiographic features (p. 52) that help to distinguish between a fracture and a vessel marking.
- The normal sphenoid sinus.
  - In young children it is not pneumatised.
  - In adults it contains air. The variable pneumatisation causes the radiographic appearance to differ widely between individuals.

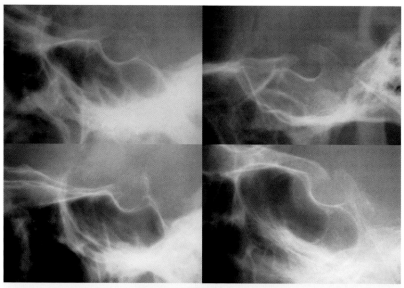

Variable appearance of the normal sphenoid sinus. Variation occurs in older children and adults because of individual differences in pneumatisation.

Analysis: recognising a fracture

In practice, the detection of a SXR abnormality is easy. There are really only three findings/abnormalities that indicate that a fracture is present—and one of these is very rare. The radiographs need to be checked/inspected in a systematic manner.

Step 1

Scrutinise the area on the radiograph which corresponds to the site of injury. Vary the windowing if necessary.

Step 2

Look for three abnormalities:

- Linear fracture. A lucent (black) line.

- Depressed fracture. A dense white area or parallel white lines due to overlapping or rotated bone fragments.

- Fluid level in the sphenoid sinus. This will be visible on the lateral film since the radiograph is taken using a horizontal X-ray beam. A fluid level indicates haemorrhage or cerebrospinal fluid within the sinus and suggests that a base of skull fracture is present. In practice a sphenoid sinus fluid level is a rare finding, but it may be the only abnormality on the radiograph.

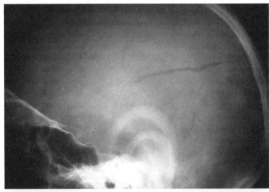

Linear fracture.

Fracture through the parietal bone.

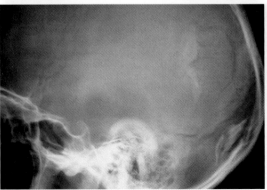

Depressed fracture.

Extensive parieto-occipital fracture with both linear (black) and depressed (white) components.

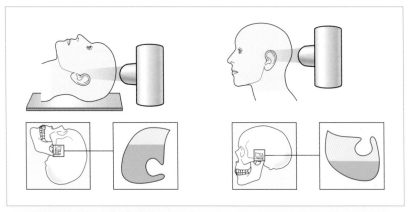

The appearance of a fluid level in the sphenoid sinus will depend on the position of the patient. It is important to know how the patient's lateral view has been obtained.

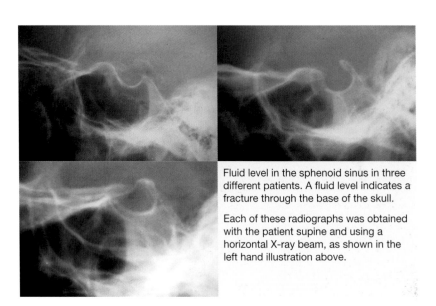

Fluid level in the sphenoid sinus in three different patients. A fluid level indicates a fracture through the base of the skull.

Each of these radiographs was obtained with the patient supine and using a horizontal X-ray beam, as shown in the left hand illustration above.

A frequent pitfall

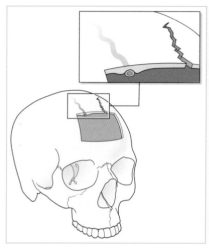

Vascular marking versus fracture.

Vascular markings appear grey because the vessel lies in a groove and consequently only the inner table of the skull is thinned. Vascular markings also have branches that gradually decrease in size as the vessel extends peripherally. Vessels have well-defined margins that are white (sclerotic).

In contrast, a fracture will often appear as a black line, because the inner and outer tables of the skull have been breached. It may have branches (ie radiating fracture lines), but these will not taper in a uniform manner and the margins of a branch will not be sclerotic.

References

1. Head injury: Triage, assessment, investigation and early management of head injury in infants, children and adults. NICE Clinical guideline 56, 2007.
2. The Royal College of Radiologists. iRefer: Making the best use of clinical radiology. London. The Royal College of Radiologists, 2012.
3. Management of minor head injury in children. Letter from the Chief Medical Officer, Northern Ireland 2005. Ref: HSS(MD) 11/2005.
4. Reed MJ, Browning JG, Wilkinson AG, Beattie T. Can we abolish skull Xrays for head injury? Arch Dis Child 2005; 90: 859–864.
5. Stiell IG, Clement CM, Rowe BH et al. Comparison of the Canadian CT Head Rule and the New Orleans Criteria in Patients with Minor Head Injury. JAMA 2005; 294: 1511–1518.
6. Glauser J. Head Injury: Which patients need imaging? Which test is best? Cleveland Clin J Med 2004; 71: 353–357.
7. Moseley I. Skull fractures and mild head injury. J Neurol Neurosurg Psychiatry 2000; 68: 403–404.
8. Hofman PA, Nelemans P, Kemerink GJ, Wilmink JT. Value of radiological diagnosis of skull fracture in the management of mild head injury: meta-analysis. J Neurol Neurosurg Psychiatry 2000; 68: 416–422.
9. SIGN Guideline No. 110. Early management of adult patients with a head injury. Scottish Intercollegiate Guidelines Network. ISBN 978 1 905813 46 9 May 2009.

5 Face

Normal anatomy: midface & orbit

Normal anatomy: mandible

Analysis: the checklists

The common injuries

Pitfalls

The standard radiographs[1–9]

Midface and Orbit: one or two **OM views**; occasionally with a **lateral view**.

Mandible: **OPG**, preferably with a **PA view**.

Regularly overlooked injuries

- Tripod fracture.
- Blow-out fracture.
- TMJ dislocation.
- Mandibular condyle fracture.

Abbreviations

CT, computed tomography;
OM, occipitomental view;
OM15/OM30, OM views with 15° or 30° of angulation of the X-ray beam;
OPG, orthopantomogram;
PA, posterior-anterior;
TMJ, temporomandibular joint.

Normal anatomy: midface & orbit

Facial bone anatomy

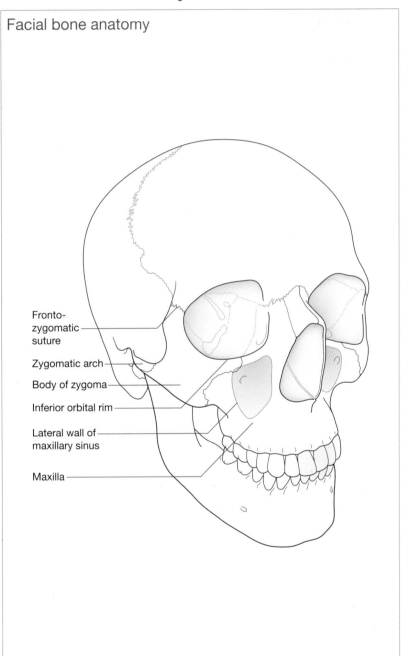

Fronto-
zygomatic
suture

Zygomatic arch

Body of zygoma

Inferior orbital rim

Lateral wall of
maxillary sinus

Maxilla

Occipitomental (OM) views

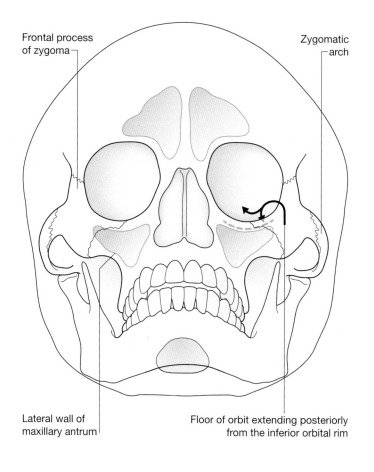

Frontal process
of zygoma

Zygomatic
arch

Lateral wall of
maxillary antrum

Floor of orbit extending posteriorly
from the inferior orbital rim

Normal anatomy: mandible

The orthopantomogram (OPG)

The OPG is a technique for demonstrating the mandible, temporomandibular joints and teeth in a single plane. The X-ray tube and the film cassette rotate around the patient and the exposure lasts a few seconds. A panoramic image is obtained.

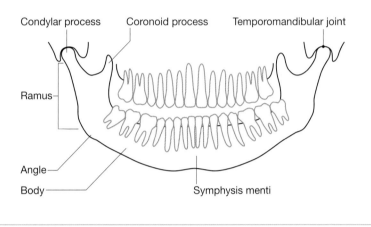

The temporomandibular joint (TMJ)

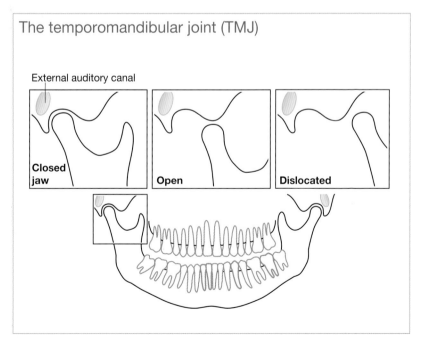

Straight PA radiograph

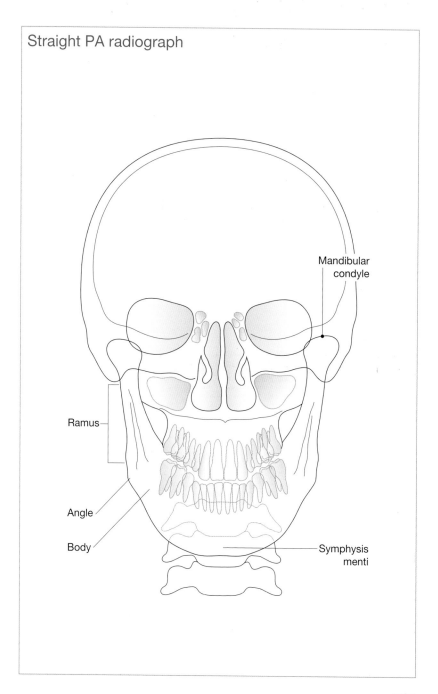

Mandibular condyle

Ramus

Angle

Body

Symphysis menti

Analysis: the checklists

Midface injury

The midface anatomy appears very complex. Try this approach. Think of the zygoma (malar bone) as a midface stool with four legs. The seat of the stool is very strong. The four legs are much weaker, so you need to assess each leg very carefully.

A five-point checklist

Inspect the OM views as follows:

Concentrate on the stool's legs. For each leg compare the injured side with the other (normal) side. Look for any asymmetry or any difference between the appearance of the matching legs. Check as follows:

1. Leg 1: zygomatic arch.

2. Leg 2: frontal process of the zygoma.

3. Leg 3: orbital floor/rim.

4. Leg 4: lateral wall of the maxillary antrum.

5. Look for fractures and look for:

   ❏ a fluid level (blood from a fracture) in the maxillary antrum;

   ❏ sinus air in the soft tissues or in the orbit.

Always apply this rule: If any one of the legs is fractured then always, always, double check whether the other three legs of the midface stool are intact (see Tripod fracture, p. 63).

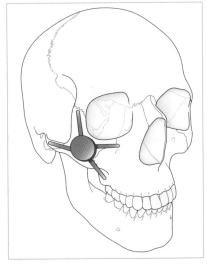 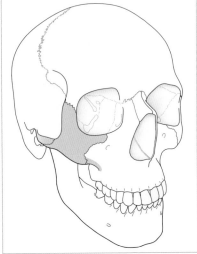

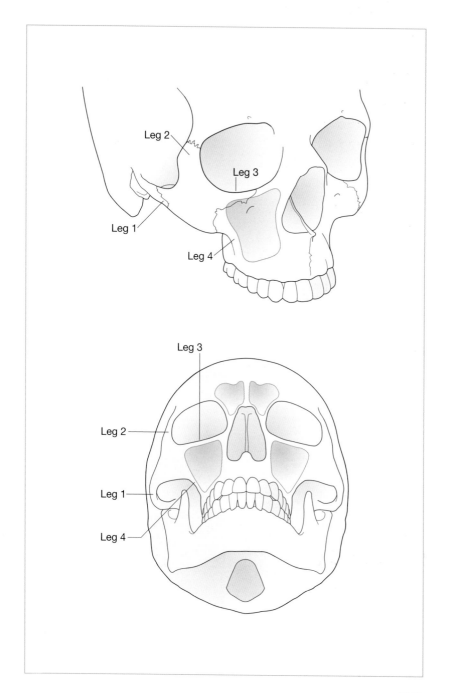

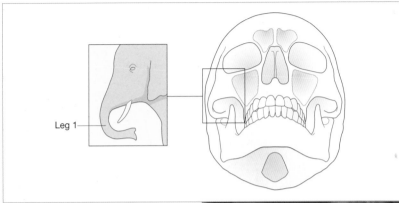

Midface stool—Leg 1

The zygomatic arch. The arch is easy to identify on the OM view, where it may be likened to an elephant's trunk. This is a frequent site of fracture, either as an isolated injury or as part of a tripod fracture. This radiograph is normal.

Potential pitfall: The normal elephant's trunk often has a normal developmental bump on its inferior surface, about half way along the trunk.

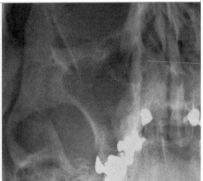

Midface stool—Legs 2 & 3

- Leg 2: frontal process of zygoma (arrow). The normal frontozygomatic suture will often be lucent. Compare this lucency with the uninjured side.

- Leg 3: orbital floor (arrowheads). This leg is slightly peculiar—it runs backwards and posteriorly from the rim of the orbit.

Normal radiograph.

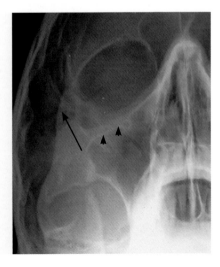

Midface stool — Leg 4

Lateral wall of the maxillary antrum (arrow).

Normal radiograph.

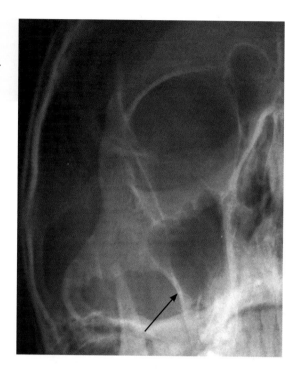

Why we do not refer to Le Fort fracture patterns

Fractures of the middle third of the face are often classified according to the Le Fort fracture patterns[3,4,10–13]. This is a useful classification for the maxillofacial surgeon when planning treatment. However, the Le Fort patterns are not particularly helpful when carrying out a step-by-step assessment of the plain radiographs in the Emergency Department. This is because the Le Fort patterns involve the pterygoid plates and the precise detail is only reliably provided by a CT scan with reconstruction of the CT images[13]. Designating a precise Le Fort injury pattern (if present) is at best guesswork when assessing plain radiographs.

Suspected blow-out fracture

Evaluate the OM view (see p. 66).

Injury to mandible

Evaluate the OPG view (see pp. 68–70).

The common injuries

Casemix varies by hospital type.

Emergency Department serving a general hospital

- Principally saturday night bar room brawling.

- Mainly nasal bone and mandible injuries. Fewer midface fractures.

Major centre receiving and treating high velocity blunt trauma[4]

- Principally high impact motor vehicle accidents.

- Mainly midface tripod fractures. Fewer nasal bone injuries.

Injuries to the midface

Isolated fracture of the zygomatic arch.

This is a common injury (arrow).

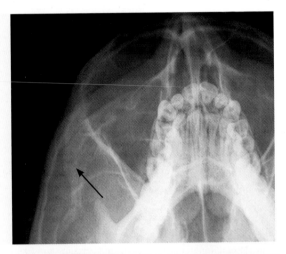

Fracture of the inferior orbital margin.

This may occur in isolation or may occur as part of a tripod fracture. An isolated rim fracture (arrow) usually involves the inferior and lateral aspect of this thick, strong, bone.

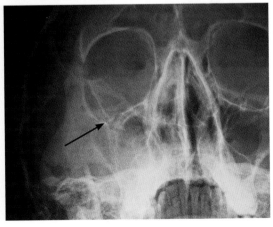

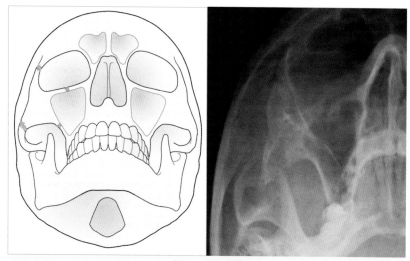

Tripod fracture. In this combination injury the cheekbone (ie the zygoma) is detached from its four points of attachment to the rest of the facial skeleton[3].

A tripod fracture comprises:

- fracture through the zygomatic arch (leg 1 of the four-legged stool)

- widening (diastasis) of the zygomaticofrontal suture (leg 2)

- fracture through the inferior orbital rim (leg 3)

- fracture through the lateral wall of the maxillary antrum (leg 4).

Arguably it would be more accurate to call it a quadripod fracture[4,13].

The Tripod fracture is also known as: Zygomaticomaxillary fracture complex; Zygomaticofacial fracture; and Trimalar fracture[3].

Tripod or quadripod? Terminological discord

The term "tripod fracture" is accepted common usage, derived from an analogy to a three legged stool to describe the midface anatomy[3,4,14]. We agree with Daffner[4] that there are really four legs supporting the stool (the zygoma), so we evaluate the four legs (pp. 58–59). Some other authors envisage a three legged stool as follows:

- The malar eminence of the zygomatic bone (the cheek bone) is regarded as the seat of a stool[3,4,14].

- The three legs are: (1) the zygomatic arch running backwards; (2) the fronto-zygomatic process running upwards; (3) the maxillary process running anteriorly and medially. This third leg is visualised as a somewhat splayed and hollowed out structure[4] forming the floor of the orbit as well as the lateral wall of the maxillary antrum.

Face

Orbital blow-out fracture

Following blunt trauma, this injury may be isolated, or accompany any other major or minor facial injury[13]. It results from a direct compressive force to the globe (ie the eyeball), commonly from a fist, elbow, dashboard, car seat, or small object such as a squash ball.

The diameter of the object that compresses the eyeball is invariably greater than the diameter of the eyeball itself. The blow causes a sudden increase in the intraorbital pressure behind the eyeball, resulting in a fracture or fractures of the thin and delicate plates of bone that form the floor and the medial wall of the orbit.

Approximately 20–40% of patients with an orbital floor blow-out fracture also have a fracture of the medial wall of the orbit[15].

Clinical impact guidelines

▦ Imaging for a suspected orbital blow-out fracture: only patients with a clear clinical indication for surgery require imaging[16]. Ultrasound evaluation is generally preferable to radiography.

▦ If some of the orbital contents herniate downwards through the orbital floor then the inferior rectus muscle may become tethered. Tethering will result in diplopia/opthalmoplegia.

▦ Decisions regarding the need for surgery revolve around:

   ❏ muscle entrapment causing opthalmoplegia

   ❏ enopthalmos.

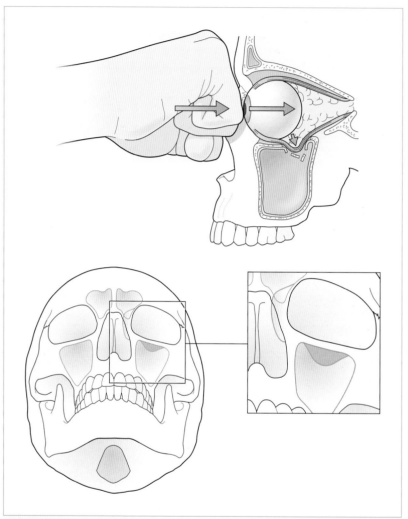

Isolated blow-out fracture.

The blow to the eyeball has increased the intraorbital pressure and resulted in a fracture of the thin plate of bone that forms the floor of the orbit. The soft tissue teardrop in the roof of the maxillary antrum represents herniated orbital contents (dark shading). Herniation through the medial wall of the orbit into the ethmoid sinus (light shading) commonly occurs but is difficult to detect on a radiograph.

Face

Orbital blow-out fracture—the OM findings

■ The strong inferior orbital margin remains intact when a blow-out fracture is an isolated injury.

■ Some orbital contents (fat and/or the inferior rectus muscle) may herniate downwards through the delicate orbital floor. This appearance has been likened to an opaque teardrop hanging from the roof of the maxillary antrum[1]. This teardrop may be the only radiographic evidence of a blow-out fracture.

■ The bone fragment (from the orbital floor) is very thin and is rarely seen.

■ Sometimes a blow-out fracture may be inferred because air from the breached sinus has entered the orbit. This orbital emphysema may be positioned above the eyeball. Air appears black on the radiograph. This has given rise to the description of the "black eyebrow" sign.

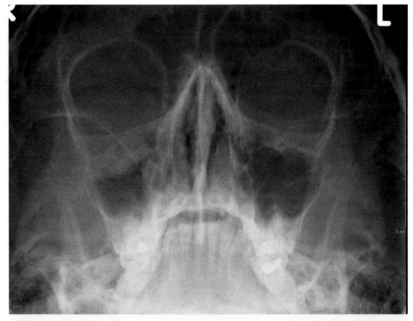

Blow-out fracture with a teardrop. Soft tissue can be seen hanging from the roof of the right maxillary antrum.

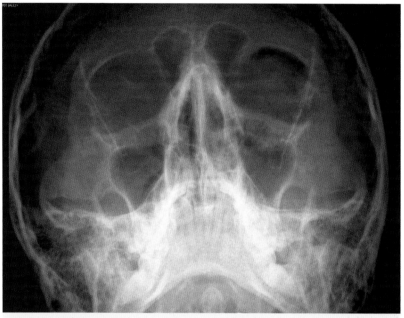

Blow-out fracture with a black eyebrow. Note the black eyebrow sign above the left eyeball. Also note the teardrop in the roof of the antrum.

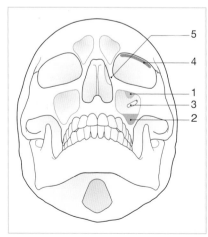

Isolated blow-out fractures. All, some or none of the following may be visible:

(1) Tear drop in antrum.

(2) Fluid level in antrum.

(3) Thin plate of bone from the orbital floor displaced into the antrum.

(4) Black eyebrow sign.

(5) Opaque (blood filled) ethmoid sinus.

Face

Injuries to the mandible

Assessing the OPG

Sometimes the panoramic view (OPG) fails to show a fracture[17]. It is very important that radiological evaluation of the mandible is correlated with the precise site of clinical concern. The symphysis is particularly difficult to evaluate on an OPG; a near normal appearance may occur when fragments override each other. Clinical suspicion must always take precedence over a seemingly normal OPG. If there is any doubt, then additional radiography is indicated—a PA radiograph in the first instance.

Important points to check

- Think of the mandible as a rigid ring of bone. When a ring of bone is broken it is very common for two fractures to occur in the ring. 50% of mandible fractures are bilateral[18].

- Always check for symmetry—compare one side of the mandible with the other.

- Check for fractures of the body and angle of the mandible.

- Assess the mandibular condyles carefully. Fractures here may be very subtle.

- Check for correct dental occlusion. The upper and lower teeth should have even and equal spacing on the radiograph. Displaced fractures, or a fracture through the neck of a condyle, frequently produce uneven spacing between the teeth[4,11].

- Check for any step deformity in the line of the teeth of the lower jaw. This invariably indicates a fracture.

- Assess the temporomandibular joint (TMJ, see p. 56).

Be careful. The OPG will produce some appearances that can be confused with a fracture. These artefacts are mainly due to the overlapping image of the pharynx or tongue. Familiarity with the possible artefacts (pp. 69 and 72) will prevent an incorrect interpretation.

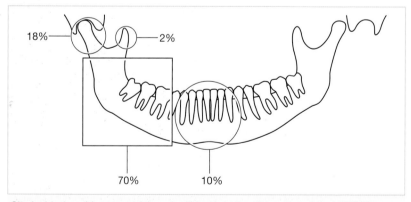

18% — 2%

70% — 10%

Site incidence of fractures of the mandible. Note the dislocation of the left TMJ.

OPG.

Two mandible fractures (arrows).

Note: in the OPGs on this page we have excluded the TMJs for illustrative purposes.

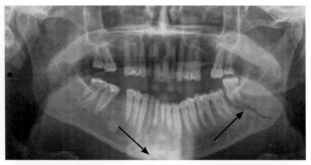

OPG.

Uneven spacing between the upper and lower teeth suggests a mandible fracture.

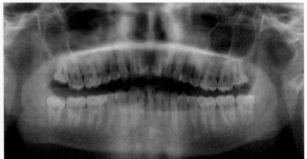

OPG.

Step deformity in the line of the lower teeth at the site of the mandible fracture.

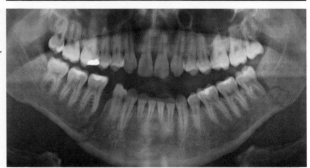

OPG.

Normal, showing artefact due to the tongue (arrows).

Occasionally an artefact may be misinterpreted as a fracture.

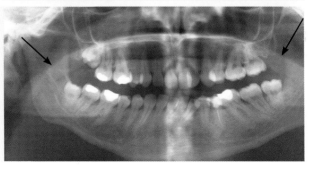

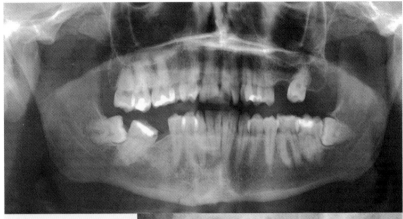

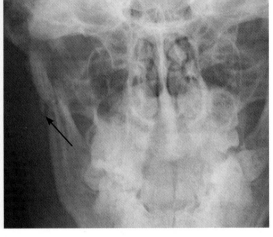

OPG and PA views.

The OPG does not readily show a fracture, but the PA does (arrow).

Helpul hint:

If the integrity of the mandible's symphysis remains equivocal following careful scrutiny of both the OPG and PA views then an occlusal radiograph (ie an intraoral image often used in routine dentistry) will provide excellent detail of this particular area.

Injuries to the nasal bone

Referral for radiography is not necessary[5,6] even if a fracture is certain on clinical examination. Radiography is only indicated when requested by a specialist surgeon.

Pitfalls

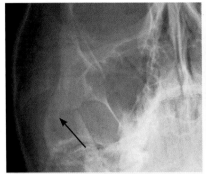

Normal bump (arrow) on the inferior aspect of a zygomatic arch. A common normal variant—a muscular attachment.

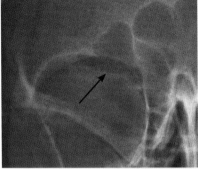

Frontal sinus extension into the orbital plate of the frontal bone (arrow) can mimic the Black Eyebrow Sign.

Eyelid trapped air (normal) mimicking a black eyebrow (arrow).

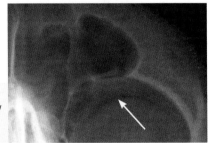

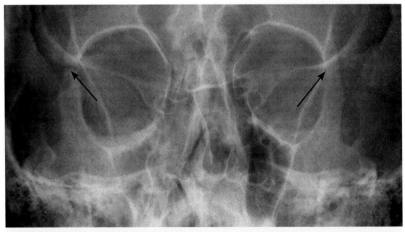

Asymmetry of the normal zygomaticofrontal sutures on an OM (arrows). This is an occasional normal variant.

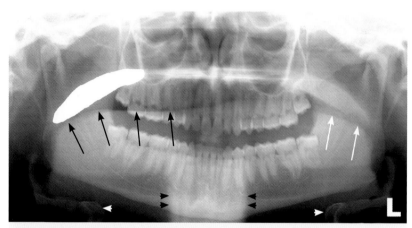

The common artefacts/normal shadows on an OPG radiograph.

Soft palate (white shaded area). Dorsal surface of the tongue (black arrows). The oropharyngeal airway between the soft palate and the dorsal surface of the tongue creates a black line across the ramus of the mandible (white arrows). The band of increased density projected over the midline is due to the cervical spine which lies outside the focal plane (black arrowheads). Hyoid bone (white arrowheads).

References

1. Perry M, Dancey A, Mireskandari K et al. Emergency care in facial trauma—a maxillofacial and ophthalmic perspective. Injury 2005; 36: 875–896.
2. Perry M. Maxillofacial trauma – developments, innovations and controversies. Injury 2009; 40: 1252–1259.
3. Dolan KD, Jacoby CG, Smoker WRK. The radiology of facial fractures. Radiographics 1984; 4: 577–663.
4. Daffner RH. Imaging of facial trauma. Curr Probl Diagn Radiol 1997; 26: 155–184.
5. de Lacey GJ, Wignall BK, Hussain S, Reidy JR. The radiology of nasal injuries: problems of interpretation and clinical relevance. Br J Radiol 1977; 50: 412–414.
6. Li S, Papsin B, Brown DH. Value of nasal radiographs in nasal trauma management. J Otolaryngol 1996; 25: 162–164.
7. Raby N, Moore D. Radiography of facial trauma, the lateral view is not required. Clin Radiol 1998; 53: 218–220.
8. McGhee A, Guse J. Radiography for midfacial trauma: is a single OM15 degrees radiograph as sensitive as OM15 degrees and OM30 degrees combined? Br J Radiol 2000; 73: 883–885.
9. Pogrel MA, Podlesh SW, Goldman KE. Efficacy of a single occipitomental radiograph to screen for midfacial fractures. J Oral Maxillofacial Surg 2000; 58: 24–26.
10. Walton RL, Hagan KF, Parry SH et al. Maxillofacial trauma. Surg Clin North Am 1982; 62: 73–96.
11. The Face. In Chan O (ed). ABC of Emergency Radiology. 3rd ed. Willey Blackwell, 2013.
12. Salvolini U. Traumatic injuries: imaging of facial injuries. Eur Radiol 2002; 12: 1253–1261.
13. Hopper RA, Salemy S, Sze RW. Diagnosis of Midface Fractures with CT: What the Surgeon needs to know. RadioGraphics 2006; 26: 783–793.
14. Rutherford WH, Illingworth R, Marsden AK et al (eds). Accident and Emergency Medicine. 2nd Ed. Edinburgh: Churchill Livingstone, 1989.
15. Dolan KD, Jacoby CG. Facial fractures. Semin Roentgenol 1978; 13: 37–51.
16. Bhattacharya J, Moseley IF, Fells P. The role of plain radiography in the management of suspected orbital blow-out fractures. Brit J Radiol 1997; 70: 29–33.
17. Druelinger L, Guenther M, Marchand EG. Radiographic evaluation of the facial complex. Emerg Med Clin North Am 2000; 18: 393–410.
18. Pathria MN, Blaser SI. Diagnostic imaging of craniofacial fractures. Rad Clin North Am 1989; 27: 839–853.

6

Shoulder

Regularly overlooked injuries

- **Dislocations/subluxations:** ACJ subluxation; complete rupture of the CC ligaments; posterior dislocation of humeral head.

- **Fractures:** scapula blade; glenoid rim or humeral head as a complication of an anterior dislocation at the GH joint.

The standard radiographs

AP view and a second view (see p. 74).

Abbreviations

ACJ, acromioclavicular joint;
AP, anterior-posterior;
CC, coracoclavicular;
GH, glenohumeral;
SC, sternoclavicular;
Y projection (view), scapula "Y" lateral.

Standard radiographs

Shoulder injury:

- The AP view is standard in all departments.

- The precise second view will vary.

  - We prefer the apical oblique projection (aka Modified Trauma Axial, MTA; see p. 76), because it allows gentle positioning of the patient, provides excellent demonstration of dislocations and shows fractures extremely well[1,2].

  - Second best: the scapula Y lateral (see p. 77). The patient is comfortable as the arm is not moved, and a true scapula Y lateral will show posterior dislocations[3]. But this view must be technically very precise, and fractures can be difficult to identify.

  - The axial (armpit) view is not recommended. It will show a posterior dislocation and most fracture fragments, but it requires abduction of the injured arm which can be very painful. It can also cause further damage. Frequently it results in a poor radiograph.

Suspected fracture of the clavicle:

- Common practice: a single AP view.

- Some departments add an additional AP with the beam angled 15° upwards.

Note our descriptive emphasis in this chapter

We are strong advocates that the second view for an injured shoulder should be the apical oblique radiograph rather than any alternative second view. Consequently, our descriptions concentrate mainly on the AP view and the apical oblique view of the injured shoulder.

Normal anatomy

AP view

The normal humeral head does not appear round and symmetrical. Its shape mimics the head of an old fashioned walking stick. This is due to the radiographer positioning the humerus in external rotation.

The articular surfaces of the glenoid and the humerus parallel one another.

The inferior cortex of the lateral part of the clavicle aligns with the inferior cortex of the acromion process. There is no step between these cortices.

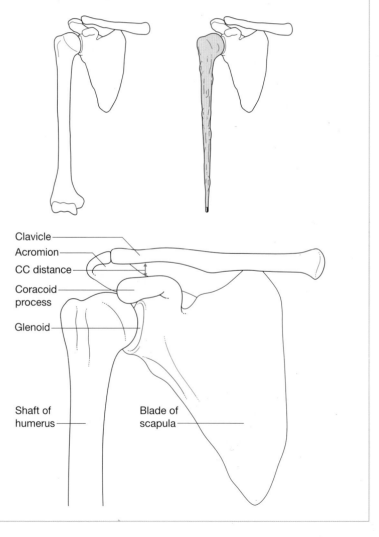

Clavicle

Acromion

CC distance

Coracoid process

Glenoid

Shaft of humerus

Blade of scapula

Apical oblique view[1,2]

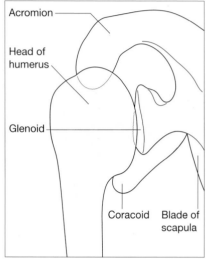

Acromion

Head of humerus

Glenoid

Coracoid   Blade of scapula

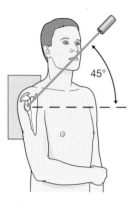

45°

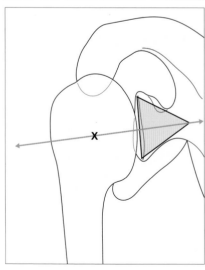

X

The normal GH joint.

- A line drawn through the apex and the centre of the base of the (imaginary) cone should pass through the centre of the humeral head.

- On this projection, anterior is downwards and posterior is upwards, as shown in the top right drawing.

Lateral scapula view—ie the Y view[3]

The humeral head overlies the centre of the glenoid. The Y is formed by the junction of the scapular blade, the coracoid and the spine of the scapula. On this view anterior is towards the ribs and posterior is away from the ribs.

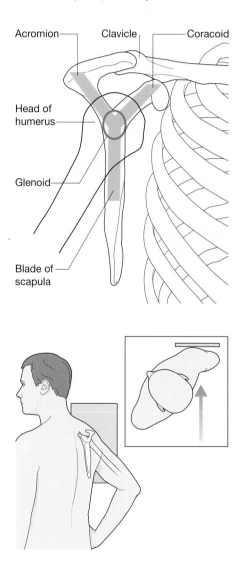

Analysis: the checklists

The AP radiograph

Ask yourself five questions.

1. Is the humeral head lying directly below the coracoid process?

    Yes = anterior dislocation.

2. Does the humeral head have a walking stick shape, and does its articular surface parallel the glenoid margin?

    No = use the second view to rule out a posterior dislocation.

3. Is the acromioclavicular joint normal—ie do the inferior cortices of the clavicle and acromion process align?

    No = subluxation or dislocation at the acromioclavicular joint.

4. Is the coracoclavicular distance more than 1.3 cm?

    Yes = stretching or rupture of the coracoclavicular ligaments (see p. 86).

5. Is there a fracture of the head or neck of the humerus, the glenoid margin, the clavicle, the body or neck of the scapula, or a rib fracture?

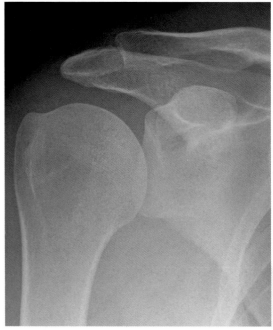

Normal shoulder.

Apply the five questions to this radiograph.

Apical oblique view[1,2]

Ask yourself three questions.

1. Do the articular surfaces of humerus and glenoid lie immediately adjacent to each other—ie does the centre of the triangle base line up with the centre of the glenoid articular surface?

    No = a glenohumeral joint dislocation or subluxation.

2. Is there a fracture of the head or the neck of the humerus?

3. Is there a fracture of the glenoid margin?

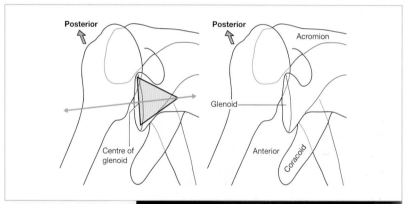

The apical oblique view is excellent in demonstrating a posterior dislocation at the glenohumeral joint.

This radiograph shows a posterior dislocation. The two drawings illustrate how an inexperienced observer can readily detect the abnormal alignment on the radiograph.

See p. 76 for the expected normal alignment on an apical oblique view.

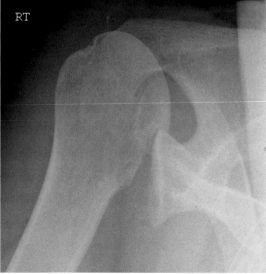

The common fractures[4–9]

Greater tuberosity of the humerus

Often undisplaced and is then very subtle (arrow). Examine the AP view very carefully.

Occasionally these fractures are invisible on the plain radiographs.

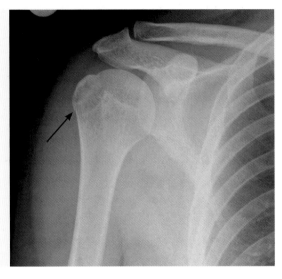

Humeral head and/or rim of the glenoid

A recognised complication of an anterior dislocation.

This apical oblique view shows the abnormal articular surface of the humeral head with a fragment (arrowhead) adjacent to it; a defect in the rim of the glenoid is also present (arrow). The glenohumeral articulation is normal.

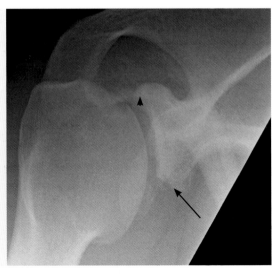

Clavicle

Accounts for 35% of all fractures involving the shoulder region[6].

- Fractures of the mid third account for 85% of clavicular fractures. Most of these occur in patients less than 20 years old. Lateral third fractures occur less frequently, and mainly in adults.

- In young children, a Greenstick fracture may occur (pp. 18–19), and appears as a slight kink in the bone.

- **Clinical impact guideline:** a clavicle fracture in an infant is a recognised complication of traumatic birth delivery; be careful not to misdiagnose this finding as a non-accidental injury.

Fracture of the middle third of the clavicle.

Most mid third fractures occur as a result of a fall on the shoulder. Some result from a transmitted force (ie a fall on the outstretched hand).

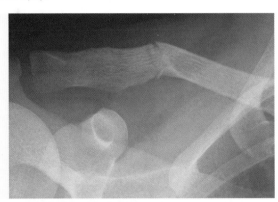

Fracture of the lateral third of the clavicle.

Often due to a direct blow to the clavicle (eg during a contact sport, a fall, or a road traffic accident).

Clinical impact guideline: more likely than a middle third fracture to be associated with delayed union or non union[10].

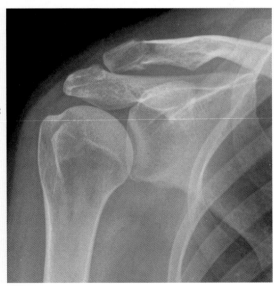

The common dislocations[4,8,9]

Anterior dislocation of the glenohumeral (GH) joint

GH dislocations are the commonest traumatic dislocations of the skeleton. Anterior dislocations represent 95% of all GH dislocations. The appearances shown here are characteristic and on the whole the diagnosis is straightforward.

Anterior GH dislocations are often accompanied by fractures of the greater tuberosity of the humerus: see p. 80.

Anterior dislocation of GH joint: AP view.

The head of the humerus is displaced medially (towards the ribs). In the majority of cases it lies below the coracoid process.

Essential: The second view needs to be scrutinised for:

- confirmation

- fractures

- detached fragments.

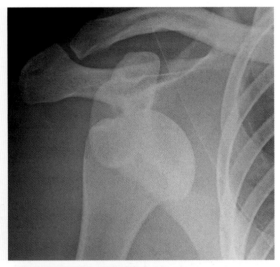

Anterior dislocation of GH joint: Apical oblique view.

The head of the humerus is seen well away from the glenoid articular surface and positioned anteriorly.

When you draw in the glenoid cone or triangle (see p. 76), the line passing through the apex of the triangle does not pass through the centre of the head of the humerus.

A bonus from an apical oblique view: exquisite visualisation of bones and articular surfaces.

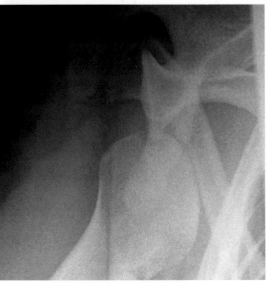

Anterior dislocation of GH joint: Scapula Y view.

The humeral head (arrows) does not cover the glenoid (arrowheads). The glenoid is identified as being at the junction of the three limbs of the "Y" (see p. 77).

A disadvantage of the scapula Y: fractures are often not visible.

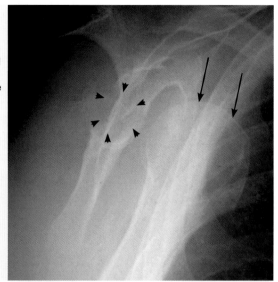

Pitfall: Haemorrhage causing subluxation.

Following an injury, usually with an intra-articular fracture, there may be extensive haemorrhage into the joint. The increase in fluid volume may push the head of the humerus inferiorly (as shown), but not medially. This inferior displacement can be misinterpreted as a dislocation.

The haemorrhage will absorb within a week or two and consequently the subluxation will resolve.

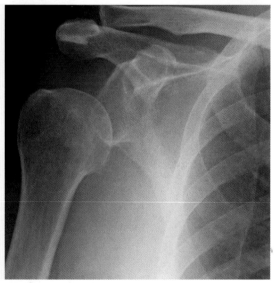

Pitfall: Hemiplegia and a subluxed humeral head

In a patient with hemiplegia, the humeral head on the affected side might not be maintained in a normal position by good muscle tone. It can drop inferiorly because the deltoid muscle is paralysed. This inferior subluxation is permanent.

Anterior dislocation of the glenohumeral (GH) joint with accompanying fractures

A fracture of the greater tuberosity of the humerus frequently accompanies a dislocation.

■ Always scrutinise both shoulder views for a fragment detached from the glenoid rim or from the posterior and superior aspect of the head of the humerus. If a fragment enters the joint it may prevent a successful reduction.

■ Compression injuries also occur: Hill–Sachs deformity and Bankart's lesion (see opposite).

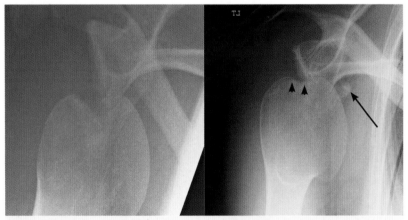

Patient (left) with a fracture of the greater tuberosity and an anterior dislocation on this apical oblique view. Patient (right) with an anterior dislocation and a fragment (arrow) detached from the head of the humerus (arrowheads).

A previous anterior dislocation had caused a fracture of the inferior margin of the glenoid (arrow).

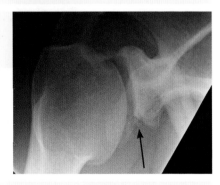

Clinical impact guideline. The post reduction radiograph must be checked to ensure that any accompanying fracture has reduced. If a fragment remains displaced it may require open reduction and internal fixation.

Hill–Sachs deformity.

A compression fracture (arrow) of the posterolateral aspect of the humeral head.

This injury results from impaction of the humeral head against the glenoid margin. It occurs in as many as 50% of anterior dislocations[7].

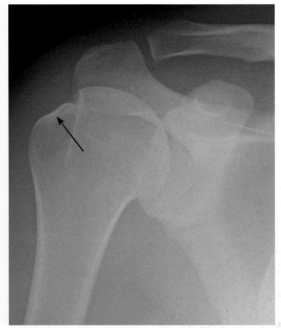

Bankart's lesion.

A fracture of the anterior lip of the glenoid.

It results from impaction by the humeral head on the glenoid during dislocation.

This apical oblique radiograph was taken following a successful reduction. The glenoid fragment is well shown inferiorly (arrow).

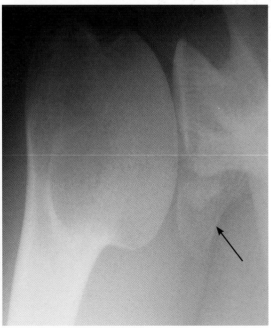

Subluxations and dislocations at the acromioclavicular joint (ACJ)

This joint is the sole bone to bone attachment of the upper limb to the rest of the skeleton.

Assess this joint on the AP view only. The other projections may mislead.

The ligaments

The coracoclavicular (CC) ligaments attach the patient's arm to the body, and prevent vertical movement of the clavicle and ACJ. The normal distance between the coracoid and clavicle on the AP view is usually less than 1.3 cm[4,5]. Complete dislocation of the ACJ indicates rupture of CC ligaments (see opposite).

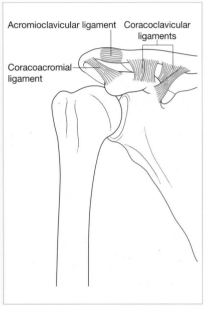

Acromioclavicular ligament   Coracoclavicular ligaments

Coracoacromial ligament

Abnormal findings:

- The inferior cortices of the clavicle and acromion do not align.

- If the CC distance is greater than 1.3 cm then rupture of the CC ligaments is probable.

Stress radiographs will help in equivocal cases of CC ligament rupture. The radiograph should ideally be obtained with the weights hanging from the wrists, in order to ensure full relaxation of the upper limb muscles.

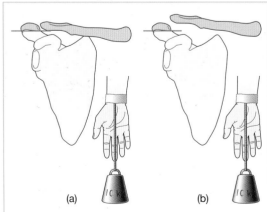

(a)   (b)

Weight bearing views.

Normal and abnormal alignment of the inferior surfaces of the acromion process and the clavicle.

(a) is normal;

(b) ACJ dislocation.

86

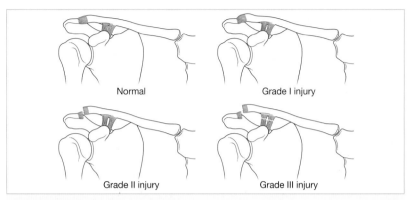

Grading the injuries to the ligaments[11].

Grade I: Stretching or partial rupture of ACJ ligament, but intact CC ligaments.
Radiological findings: normal, or slight step at ACJ.

Grade II: Rupture of ACJ ligament and stretching of CC ligaments.
Radiological findings: a step at the ACJ. May need stress views if equivocal.

Grade III: Rupture of ACJ ligament and rupture of CC ligaments.
Radiological findings: a step at the ACJ and increased CC distance (ie greater than
1.3 cm). May need stress views to show the full extent of the damage.

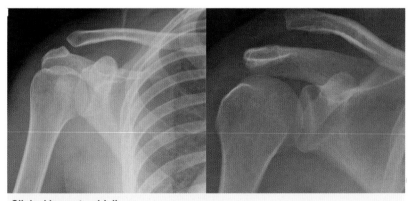

Clinical impact guidelines.

ACJ subluxation (left) is invariably treated conservatively, usually with an excellent
outcome. On the other hand, a complete ACJ dislocation (right) is an important injury.
Opinion regarding management varies. It will be treated conservatively by some
surgeons who then reserve surgery for those who develop persistent symptoms.
Other surgeons advise early surgery for nearly all ACJ dislocations, particularly for
manual workers and athletes.

Shoulder

Uncommon but important injuries

Posterior dislocation at the glenohumeral (GH) joint

The naming of this injury is arguably inaccurate. It is very rarely a complete dislocation. Despite the notable posterior displacement it is, invariably, a major subluxation.

On many occasions there will be an accompanying fracture of the anterior aspect of the humeral head.

Uncommon. Fewer than 5% of shoulder dislocations. As many as 50% are overlooked even when initial radiographs show the abnormality[7].

Often caused by violent muscle contraction; either during a convulsion or from an electric shock. Sometimes, both shoulders will dislocate simultaneously[8].

Posterior dislocation: characteristic appearances on the AP view.

The rotated and posteriorly displaced humeral head loses the normal parallelism of the articular surfaces, as in the two posterior dislocations below.

The humeral head frequently appears rounded—no longer the contour of an old fashioned walking stick. The globular contour has been likened to a light bulb or drumstick appearance (right).

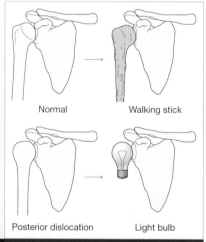

Normal   Walking stick

Posterior dislocation   Light bulb

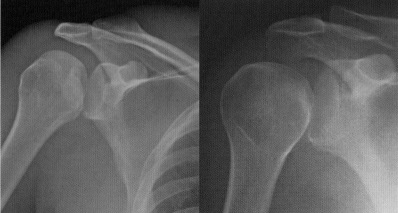

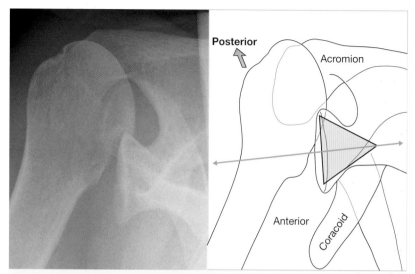

Posterior dislocation: characteristic appearances on an apical oblique view.
The main mass of the humeral head lies posterior to the glenoid.

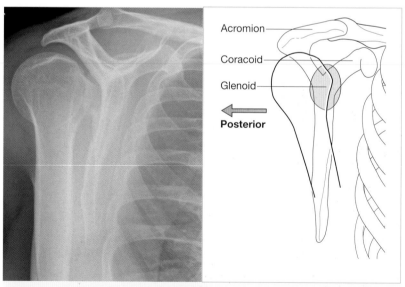

Posterior dislocation: characteristic appearance on a scapula Y view[7].
The centre of the humeral head lies posterior to the junction of the three limbs
of the Y (ie away from the ribs).

89

Fractures of the proximal humerus

Neck of humerus

Usually occurs in an osteoporotic elderly patient as a result of a fall. A greater tuberosity fracture may also be present.

In younger patients it is invariably caused by a violent force.

In children and adolescents the growth plate is involved (Salter–Harris fracture, p. 15).

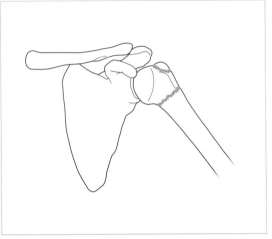

Elderly patient. Impacted fracture of the neck of the humerus.

A large joint effusion (haemorrhage) has caused the head of the humerus to sublux inferiorly.

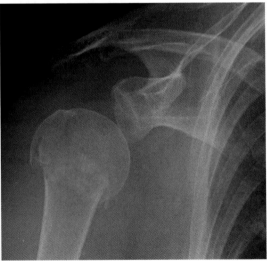

Clinical impact guidelines for fractures of the proximal humerus.

In elderly patients an impacted fracture need not be immobilised and a sling is utilised with physiotherapy and active shoulder movements. Unimpacted fractures are frequently managed with sling immobilisation.

Younger patients will usually require fracture reduction if the fragments are displaced. Sometimes a closed reduction, sometimes open reduction and internal fixation[8,9].

Fractures of the body or neck of the scapula

Usually result from a high impact event. Serious soft tissue or neurovascular injuries are recognised associations[8].

You will only see what you look for…these fractures are easy to overlook. Always check the AP and the second view very carefully.

Road traffic accident. Transverse fracture through the body of the scapula (arrows).

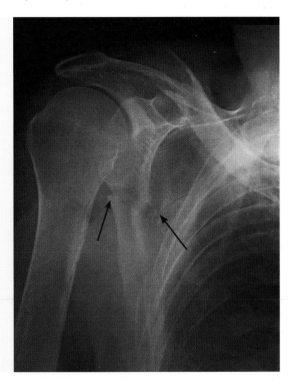

Sternoclavicular rupture

Consequent on a high impact injury. Very, very, rare. An associated vascular injury occurs in 25% of cases[4,5].

Inferior dislocation of the humeral head (luxatio erecta)

Very rare and accounts for less than 0.5% of all shoulder dislocations. The clinical finding is classical—a Statue of Liberty appearance with the arm elevated and the forearm fixed and resting on the head[5,12]. The AP radiograph shows the head of the humerus nestling immediately inferior to the glenoid with the humerus pointing upwards. Usual cause: forceful hyperabduction of an abducted limb.

Pitfalls

Positioning

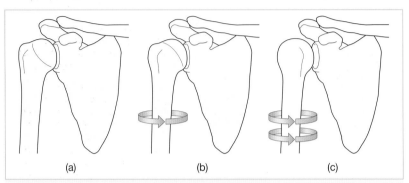

(a)	(b)	(c)

The effect of internal rotation on the contour of the humeral head. Standard AP radiographs are always obtained with the humerus positioned in slight external rotation and this accounts for the humeral head looking like a club-headed walking stick as shown in (a). However, the injured joint may be so painful that the patient holds the arm in internal rotation. When this occurs then a light bulb appearance (b,c) may result and can mimic a posterior dislocation. An error in interpretation will be avoided by checking the precise position of the humerus on the second view.

ACJ assessment

Be careful: Do not evaluate the integrity of the acromioclavicular joint (ACJ) on any of the second views. The appearance of the ACJ can be very deceptive on these projections. Always assess the ACJ on the AP radiograph alone.

Developmental variants that can mislead

On the AP view in the immature skeleton, the growth plate for the humeral head lies obliquely, appearing as two separate lines. Either of these normal lines (arrows) may be mistaken for an undisplaced fracture.

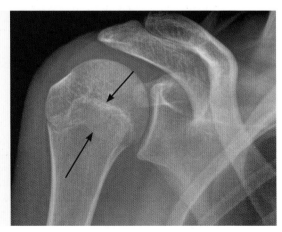

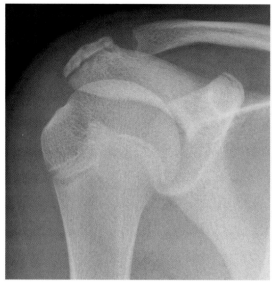

The tips of the acromion and coracoid processes ossify from separate ossification centres. In children these secondary centres may be mistaken for fracture fragments.

Occasionally the secondary centre at the tip of the acromion does not fuse with the rest of the scapula, and remains as a separate bone—the os acromiale. It may be mistaken for a fracture. Interestingly, when present, this accessory ossicle is usually bilateral.

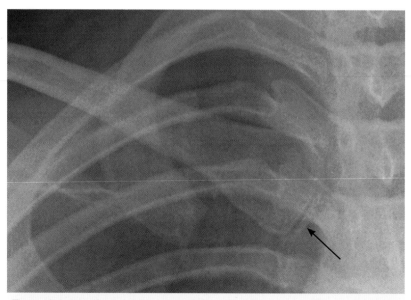

The medial clavicular epiphysis is one of the last of all the secondary centres to unite to the parent bone (at approximately 25 years of age). Do not confuse this epiphysis (arrow) with a fracture.

The rhomboid fossa.

A common normal variant. This notch or prominent depression in the inferior aspect of the medial portion of the clavicle is the point of insertion of the costoclavicular ligament attaching the clavicle to the costal cartilage of the first rib.

Do not mistake it for a pathological erosion of the clavicle.

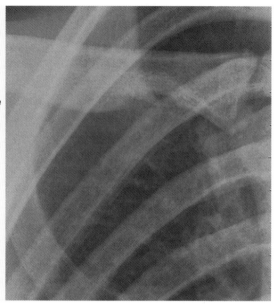

Cystic appearance: the superior and lateral aspect of the head of a normal humerus will sometimes appear lucent on a radiograph. A cyst or an area of destruction may be diagnosed erroneously.

References

1. Kornguth PJ, Salazar AM. The apical oblique view of the shoulder: its usefulness in acute trauma. Am J Roentgenol 1987; 149: 113–116.
2. Garth WP, Slappey CE, Ochs CW. Roentgenographic demonstration of instability of the shoulder: the apical oblique projection. J Bone Joint Surg 1984; 66: 1450–1453.
3. Horsfield D, Jones SN. A useful projection in radiography of the shoulder. J Bone Joint Surg 1987; 69B: 338.
4. Rogers LF. Radiology of skeletal trauma. 3rd ed. Churchill Livingstone, 2001.
5. Neustadter LM, Weiss MJ. Trauma to the shoulder girdle. Semin Roentgenol 1991; 26: 331–343.
6. Nordqvist A, Petersson CJ. Incidence and causes of shoulder girdle injuries in an urban population. J Shoulder Elbow Surg 1995; 4: 107–112.
7. The Shoulder. In Chan O (ed). ABC of Emergency Radiolgy. 3rd ed. Wiley Blackwell, 2013.
8. Hamblen DL, Simpson AH. Adams's Outline of Fractures including Joint Injuries. 12th ed. Churchill Livingstone, 2007.
9. Solomon L, Warwick DJ, Nayagam S. Apley's Concise System of Orthopaedics and Fractures. 3rd ed. Hodder Arnold, 2005.
10. Edwards DJ, Kavanagh TG, Flannery MC. Fractures of the distal clavicle; a case for fixation. Injury 1992; 23: 44–46.
11. Mlasowsky B, Brenner P, Duben W et al. Repair of complete acromioclavicular dislocation (Tossy Stage III) using Balser's hook plate combined with ligament sutures. Injury 1988; 19: 227–232.
12. Patel DN, Zuckerman JD, Egol KA. Luxatio erecta: case series with review of diagnostic and management principles. Am J Orthop 2011; 40: 566–570.

7 Paediatric elbow

Regularly overlooked injuries

- Undisplaced supracondylar fracture.
- Fracture, lateral condyle of humerus.
- Monteggia injury[1,2].

The standard radiographs

AP in full extension.
Lateral with 90 degrees of flexion.

Abbreviations

CRITOL: **C**apitellum, **R**adial head, **I**nternal epicondyle, **T**rochlea, **O**lecranon, **L**ateral epicondyle.

Anatomy

AP view—child age 9 or 10 years

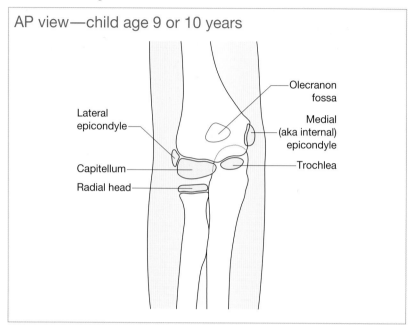

Olecranon fossa

Lateral epicondyle

Medial (aka internal) epicondyle

Capitellum

Trochlea

Radial head

Lateral view—child age 9 or 10 years

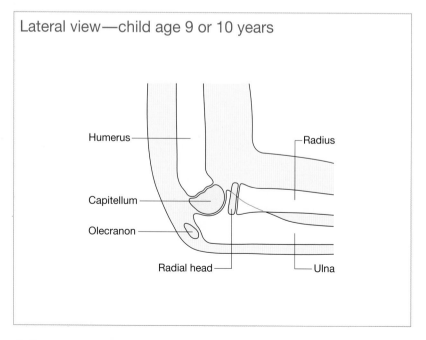

Humerus

Radius

Capitellum

Olecranon

Radial head

Ulna

Elbow fat pads

There are pads of fat close to the distal humerus, anteriorly and posteriorly. They are extrasynovial but intracapsular.

- Look for the fat pads on the lateral. They are not seen on the AP view.

- The fat is visualised as a dark streak amongst the surrounding grey soft tissues.

- The anterior fat pad is seen in most (but not all) normal elbows.
  It is closely applied to the humerus, as shown below.

- The posterior fat pad is not visible on a normal radiograph because it is situated deep within the olecranon fossa and hidden by the overlying bone.

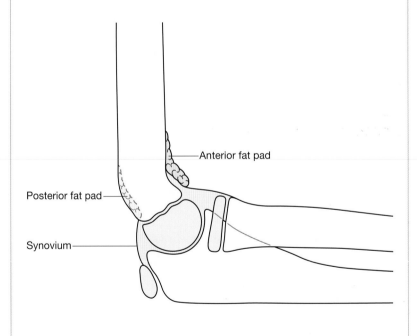

Paediatric elbow

AP and lateral: the CRITOL sequence

CRITOL: the sequence in which the ossified centres appear

At birth the ends of the radius, ulna and humerus are lumps of cartilage, and not visible on a radiograph. The large, seemingly empty, cartilage filled gap between the distal humerus and the radius and the ulna is normal.

From 6 months to 12 years the cartilaginous secondary centres begin to ossify. There are six ossification centres. Four belong to the humerus, one to the radius, and one to the ulna. Gradually the humeral centres ossify, enlarge, and coalesce. Eventually each of the fully ossified epiphyses fuses to the shaft of its particular bone.

When the ossification centres appear is not important. The order is important.

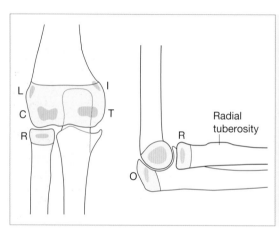

Normal ossification centres in the cartilaginous ends of the long bones.

Order of appearance from birth to 12 years:

C = capitellum
R = radial head
I = internal epicondyle
T = trochlea
O = olecranon
L = lateral epicondyle

Normal appearances are shown opposite.

Exceptions to the CRITOL sequence?

Exceptions are an occasional normal variant[3,4].

A 2011 survey[4] of 500 paediatric elbow radiographs found:

- 97% followed the CRITOL order.

- 3% showed a slightly different order.

- **But:** there were no instances in which the trochlear ossification centre appeared before the medial (internal) epicondylar centre.

Conclusions

- CRITOL is a really helpful tool when analysing a child's injured elbow.

- Occasionally a minor variation in the sequence may occur.

- Use the rule: "I always appears before T". So, if you see the ossified T before the I then the internal epicondyle has almost certainly been avulsed and is lying within the joint... ie it is masquerading as the trochlear ossification centre (see p. 105).

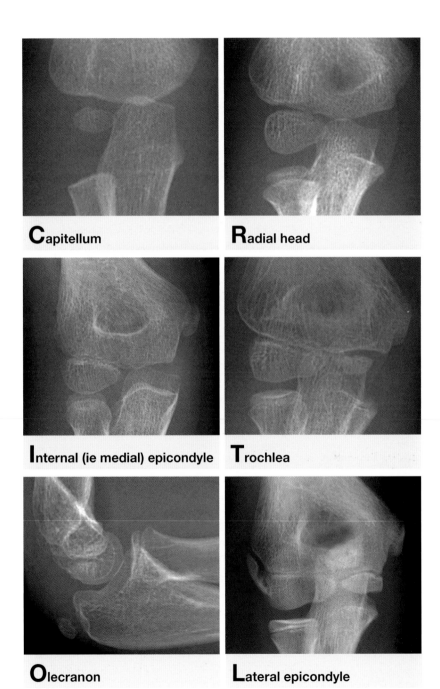

Capitellum

Radial head

Internal (ie medial) epicondyle

Trochlea

Olecranon

Lateral epicondyle

99

Paediatric elbow

Medial epicondyle—normal anatomy

Is the medial epicondyle slightly displaced/avulsed? A common dilemma.

░ **The rule to apply:**

On the AP radiograph a normally positioned epicondyle will be partly covered by some of the humeral metaphysis.

░ **A caveat:**

Occasionally a child in pain will hold the forearm in a position of slight internal rotation. Rotation will project the metaphysis of the humerus away from a normally positioned epicondyle.

░ **Conclusions:**

When checking the position of the internal epicondyle on the AP radiograph:

1. If part of the epicondyle is covered by part of the humeral metaphysis then an avulsion has not occurred.

2. A completely uncovered epicondyle indicates an avulsion... unless the forearm bones are slightly rotated.

Clinical impact guidelines: the I in CRITOL

The ossification centre for the internal (ie medial) epicondyle is the point of attachment of the forearm flexor muscles. Vigorous muscle contraction may avulse this centre (see p. 105). The most common injury mechanism is a fall on an outstretched hand. Avulsions also occur in children who are involved in throwing sports, hence the term "little leaguer's elbow".

When a major displacement of the internal epicondyle occurs the bone can become trapped within the elbow joint. This is a well recognised complication of a dislocated elbow, occurring in 50% of cases following an elbow subluxation or dislocation. A major avulsion is easy to overlook when an elbow has been transiently dislocated and then reduces spontaneously[5,6] because the detached epicondyle may, on the AP radiograph, be mistaken for the normally positioned trochlear ossification centre (p. 105).

I before T. Though the CRITOL sequence may vary slightly there is a constant: the trochlear (T) centre always ossifies after the internal epicondyle. Therefore apply this rule: if the trochlear centre (T) is visible then there must be an ossified internal epicondyle (I) visible somewhere on the radiograph. If the internal epicondyle is not seen in its normal position then suspect that it is trapped within the joint.

AP and lateral—two anatomical lines

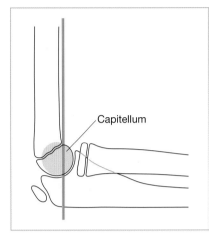

Capitellum

Anterior humeral line (on lateral).

Normal alignment: when drawn along the anterior cortex of the humerus, in most normal patients at least one third of the ossifying capitellum lies anterior to this line.

Be careful: in very young children the ossification within the cartilage of the capitellum might be minimal (ie normal and age related), and so is insufficiently calcified and does not allow application of the above rule.

This line helps you to detect a supracondylar fracture with posterior displacement (pp. 106–108).

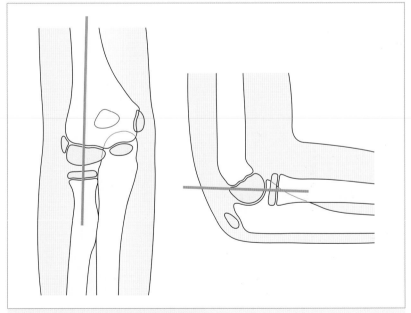

Radiocapitellar line (on AP and lateral)

Normal alignment: On the lateral radiograph a line drawn along the central axis of the proximal 2–3 cm of the radius should pass through the centre of the capitellum. If it fails to do so, the radius is dislocated at the elbow joint. The same inference can be applied to the AP view but less reliably[7].

Analysis: four questions to answer

Question 1—Are the fat pads normal?

Check the fat pads on the lateral projection.

If an effusion is present it distends the capsule, displacing the fat pads away from the bone. This provides evidence of a significant injury.

- A displaced anterior fat pad (the sail sign) is abnormal[8].

- A visible posterior fat pad is always abnormal[7]. It denotes a very large effusion —usually a considerable volume of blood in the joint.

- Not all joint effusions are associated with a fracture[8].

- An effusion indicates that a significant injury has occurred, even if a fracture is not seen. Whenever either fat pad is displaced but no fracture identified, the arm needs to be placed in a collar and cuff until orthopaedic assessment a few days later. Some of these patients will have sustained an undisplaced fracture[8,9].

- NB: Absence of a visible fat pad does not exclude a fracture. The radial neck is usually extracapsular, and a fracture of the neck may not produce a joint effusion/ haemarthrosis or displace the fat pads. Alternatively, if the joint capsule has ruptured, blood gradually leaks out of the joint into the surrounding soft tissues.

Clinical impact guidelines:
Fat pad displacement, but no fracture or dislocation identified—what to do?

It is most important that neither an undisplaced supracondylar fracture nor a displaced internal epicondyle are overlooked. The radiographs must be checked by an experienced observer before the patient is discharged.

If a fracture is still not identified then manage as for an undisplaced fracture. At clinical review in 10 days: if clinically normal—no further radiography; if clinically abnormal— obtain repeat radiographs.

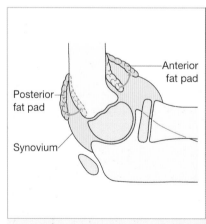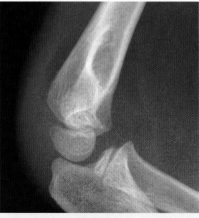

The anterior and posterior fat pads (ie the black streaks on the radiograph) are displaced by a large effusion in the elbow joint.

Question 2—Is the anterior humeral line normal?

The supracondylar region is a site of particular weakness in the developing humerus. There is a deep posterior fossa above the humeral condyles, which allows the olecranon to lie within it when the forearm is fully extended. Thus the humerus has a narrow AP diameter at this level and is a point of weakness.

The rule: A line traced along the anterior cortex of the humerus should have at least one third of the capitellum anterior to it (see p. 101).

▨　If less than one third of the capitellum lies anterior to this line, there is a strong probability of a supracondylar fracture with the distal fragment (including the capitellum) displaced posteriorly (see p. 107).

The drawing:

The capitellum is of a good size. Approximately a third of it lies in front of the anterior humeral line. Normal appearance.

The radiographs:

The abnormal anterior humeral line suggests a supracondylar fracture.

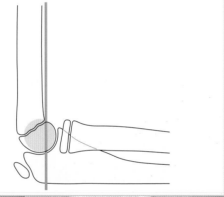

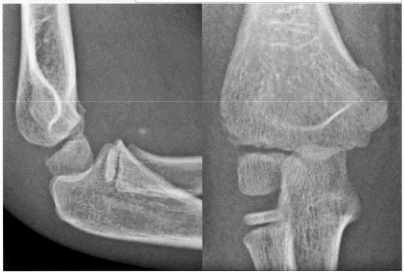

Paediatric elbow

Question 3—Is the radiocapitellar (RC) line normal?

The rule: A line drawn along the longitudinal axis of the radial head and neck should pass through the capitellum. If it does not pass through the capitellum: a radial head dislocation is likely.

- **Be careful**: the normal radius frequently shows a bend or slight angulation in the region of its tuberosity. Draw the RC line along the long axis of the proximal 2–3 cm of the radius...not along the long central axis of the shaft of the radius.

- **Be careful**: this rule is **always** valid on a true lateral[7], but on the AP radiograph the RC line can be distorted by radiographic positioning. A misleading RC line on the AP view may also be due to eccentric ossification of either the radial head or the capitellar epiphysis, which can cause the RC line to be directed away from the capitellum.

- **Be very careful**: Monteggia injury[1,2]. Whenever there is a fracture of the shaft of the ulna, evaluate the RC line carefully, because there may be an associated dislocation of the radial head. Particularly likely when there is angulation or displacement of the fracture but the radial shaft appears intact (see pp. 112–113).

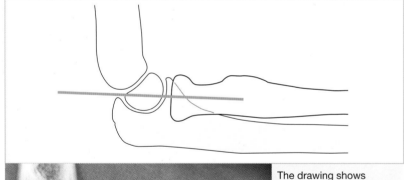

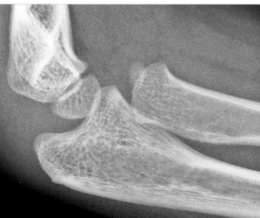

The drawing shows an elbow with a normal RC line.

The radiograph shows that a RC line would not pass through the capitellum.

Diagnosis: the radial head is dislocated.

Question 4—Are the ossification centres normal?

A most important question. Normal appearances are described on pp 96–99.

Check:

- The position of the medial epicondyle.
- The appearance of the lateral epicondyle.
- The CRITOL ossification sequence.

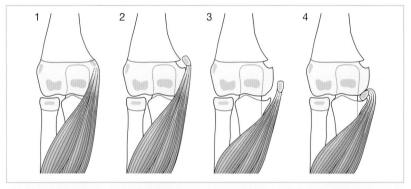

Avulsion of the internal (medial) epicondyle. 1 = normal; 2 = slight avulsion; 3 = major avulsion; 4 = major avulsion and the epicondyle lies within the joint.

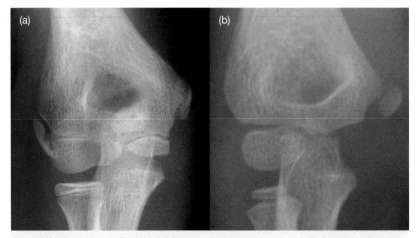

Two different patients. Both had fallen on an outstretched hand. Patient (a): normal position of the internal epicondyle. Note that the metaphysis of the humerus overlaps part of the epicondyle. Patient (b): the internal epicondyle has been avulsed. Note the lack of metaphyseal overlap.

The common injuries

Supracondylar fracture

60% of elbow fractures[9–12]. The commonest fracture in children under the age of 7 years, and the second commonest up to the age of 16 years[9].

Caused by falling on an outstretched hand with hyperextension of the elbow. The supracondylar bone is relatively thin and weak in a child.

25% of these fractures are minimally displaced or undisplaced[11,12]. Displacement is usually posterior due to the direction of the fall. Very occasionally the displacement is anterior, resulting from a blow to the posterior aspect of the elbow.

Assessment of the anterior humeral line (p. 101) is the key to recognising any posterior displacement of this fracture.

Be cautious:

▨ The anterior humeral line rule is not always reliable in very young children, due to normal but partial ossification of the capitellum.

▨ If the anterior humeral line appears abnormal and a supracondylar fracture is not identified, seek an experienced opinion.

Clinical impact guideline:

This fracture may cause vascular damage if there is major displacement. The brachial artery is situated anterior to the humeral cortex in the supracondylar region of the humerus, and can be lacerated by a bone fragment.

▨ If this fracture is displaced it needs to be reduced and stabilised to protect the vascular supply to the arm[12].

▨ Bleeding from torn vessels can also cause a compartment syndrome; ie bleeding or swelling within the adjacent muscles that are enclosed by a tight fascia. The pressure within the compartment can rise and this can cut off the blood supply to the muscles.

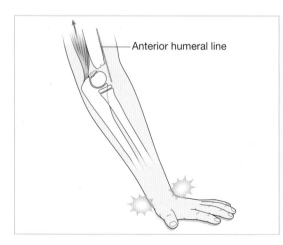

Anterior humeral line

This child has fallen on his outstretched hand and sustained a supracondylar fracture—the bone has snapped across this thin part of the humerus. The posterior displacement has occurred partly because of the resulting pull of the triceps muscle on the olecranon.

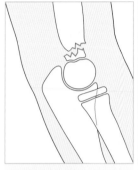

Supracondylar fracture with posterior displacement.

Very common.

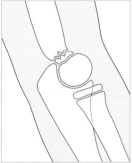

Undisplaced supracondylar fracture.

Common.

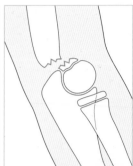

Supracondylar fracture with anterior displacement.

Uncommon.

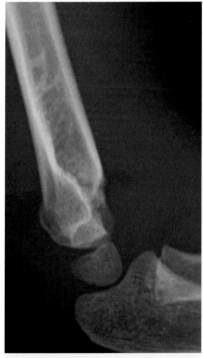

Abnormal anterior humeral line. Supracondylar fracture with posterior displacement.

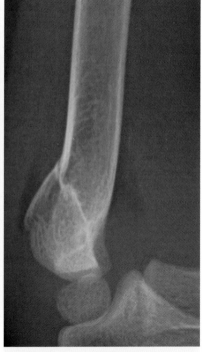

Abnormal anterior humeral line. Supracondylar fracture with posterior displacement.

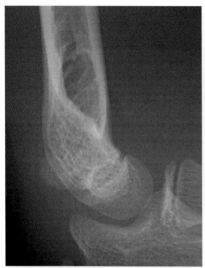

Normal elbow. The anterior humeral line is normal. Incidentally, the medial epicondyle is positioned far posteriorly. This is the normal position.

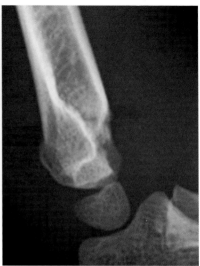

Abnormal anterior humeral line. Supracondylar fracture with posterior displacement.

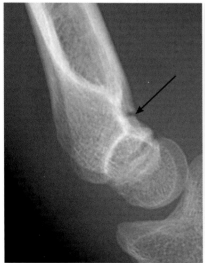

Normal anterior humeral line. Note the undisplaced supracondylar fracture (arrow).

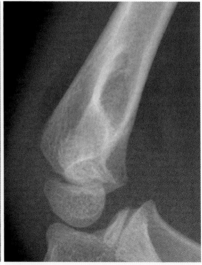

Abnormal anterior humeral line. Supracondylar fracture with posterior displacement.

Fracture of the lateral humeral condyle

The commonest fracture in children under the age of seven years. In many cases the fracture involves only the cartilaginous part of the distal humeral epiphysis. Cartilage does not show up on a radiograph. Consequently, the extensive epiphyseal component of this fracture is often not fully appreciated. In effect this is a Salter–Harris type 4 epiphyseal fracture (see p. 15).

■ Precise reduction is important If the fracture is displaced. Otherwise stiffness, cubitus valgus and/or a delayed ulnar nerve palsy may result[13].

■ **Helpful hint:** there is a recognised association between olecranon fractures and lateral condyle fractures. Have you checked the olecranon?

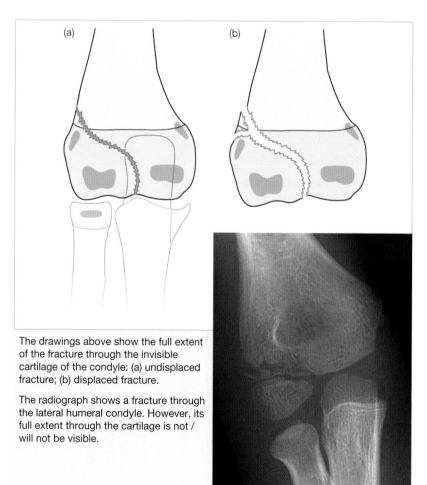

(a) (b)

The drawings above show the full extent of the fracture through the invisible cartilage of the condyle: (a) undisplaced fracture; (b) displaced fracture.

The radiograph shows a fracture through the lateral humeral condyle. However, its full extent through the cartilage is not / will not be visible.

Avulsion of the medial epicondyle

Results from a pull at the insertion of the common origins of the flexor muscles, usually as a result of a valgus stress during a fall on the outstretched hand. May also occur in throwing sports such as baseball pitching ("little leaguer's elbow").

Minor avulsion is common. The avulsed ossification centre will usually heal by fibrous union and the attachment of the flexor muscles will be stable[5,6,13]. Surgical reduction is often indicated when the avulsion is extensive, in order to obtain and preserve full function.

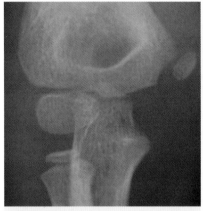

Mild/minor displacement.

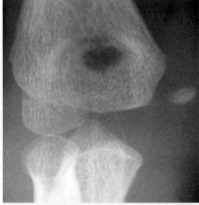

Extensive displacement.

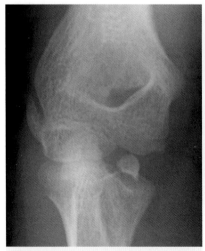

The avulsed epicondyle is situated within the elbow joint.

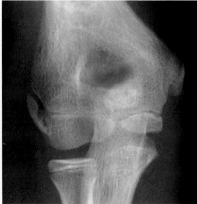

Normal position of medial epicondyle. Note the partial overlap of the epicondyle by the metaphysis of the humerus (p. 100). The other secondary centres are also normal.

Pulled ("nursemaids") elbow

Usually occurs between the age of one and four years.

Caused by a sudden jerk on the arm, often when restraining a child who is charging off to cross a busy road, or when being playfully swung around by the arm. The jerk causes the annular ligament around the head of the radius to stretch and consequently the radial head subluxes or slips very slightly.

Clinical findings are classical: the arm is held in flexion and pronation. Reduction is usually simple, quick and effective.

Radiography is not indicated as the history and clinical findings are characteristic. Also, the radiographs will always appear normal.

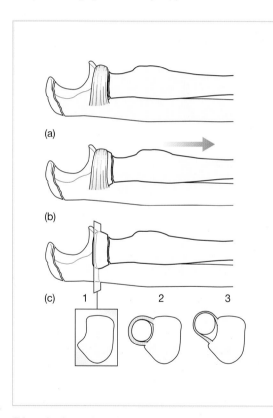

Nursemaid's elbow.

A widely held misconception is that the head of the radius subluxes distally under the annular ligament (a,b).

An ultrasound study[14] provides a different explanation (c). A cross-section at the level of the annular ligament demonstrates a shallow depression on the lateral margin of the ulna (1). The normal anatomy is shown in (2). A pulled elbow injury causes the head of the radius to perch on the anterior rim of the ulnar depression (3). This ventral subluxation explains why a successful reduction is often preceded by a snap or a click, caused by the head dropping back into its natural position.

Plastic bowing injury

In children the long bones are relatively pliable as compared with an adult and there may not be the usual ulnar or radial fracture with a visible break[2,11]. Instead, a forearm bone may bend. This is referred to as a plastic bowing injury or fracture (p. 21).

Rare but important injuries

Avulsion of the lateral epicondyle

A very rare injury. The normal elbow will often show the lateral epicondyle well away from the adjacent humeral metaphysis. This is not a cause for worry if the two adjacent cortices parallel one another (as shown on p. 113).

Isolated dislocation of the head of the radius

Abnormal radiocapitellar (RC) line (p. 101). Isolated dislocation of the radial head.

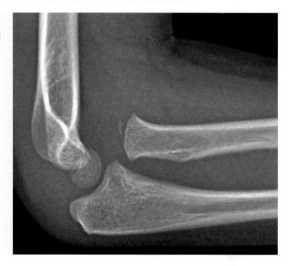

Monteggia injury

A Monteggia injury adheres to the principle of the Two Bone Rule. In a two bone system[15] such as the radius and ulna, where the bones are tightly bound together, they can be regarded as acting as a single functional unit. If one of the bones is fractured and displaced (or bent in a child) then there will need to be an additional disturbance in their relationship, often a displaced fracture of the adjacent bone. If the adjacent bone is intact then the disturbance will affect a joint. A Monteggia injury comprises a displaced fracture of the ulna (or a bowed ulna), an intact radial shaft, and a dislocated head of the radius.

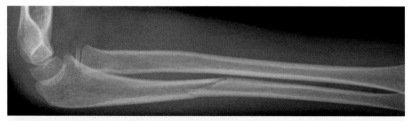

Fracture of middle third of the ulna with slight angulation.
But… the RC line is abnormal. This is a Monteggia injury.

Top: displaced fracture of the ulna. Intact radius. RC line is abnormal indicating a dislocation of the head of the radius.

Bottom: the shaft of the ulna is bent. Radial shaft is intact. RC line is abnormal.

In both cases these are Monteggia injuries.

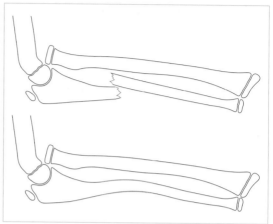

Pitfalls

Normal variants that can mislead

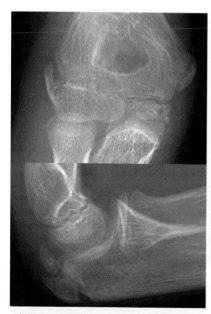

Multiple ossification centres in the trochlea and olecranon epiphyses. These are common normal variants.

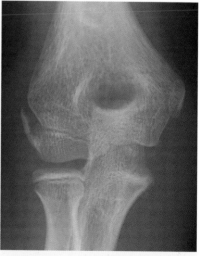

The lateral epicondyle is seemingly well away from the humerus. This is a common normal finding. Note that the epicondyle parallels the cortex of the adjacent humeral metaphysis—a characteristically normal feature.

Paediatric elbow

Puzzled by the appearance of the epicondyles?

▨ On the lateral projection do not be alarmed at seeing the medial epicondyle situated very far posteriorly (p. 108). This is its normal position.

▨ The external (ie lateral) epicondyle can be normal but seemingly widely separate from the humerus. **The rule to apply:** when normal, its lateral border is always parallel to the cortex of the adjacent humeral metaphysis (p. 112).

Misleading lines

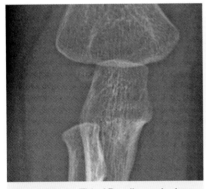

Normal elbow. This AP radiograph shows a misleading RC line (p. 104).

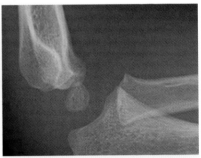

Normal elbow. This capitellum is only partly ossified (normal for age) and the anterior humeral line rule (p. 101) cannot be applied.

References

1. Dormans JP, Rang M. The problem of Monteggia fracture—dislocations in children. Orthop Clin North Am 1990; 21: 251–256.
2. David-West KS, Wilson NI, Sherlock DA et al. Missed Monteggia injuries. Injury 2005; 36: 1206–1209.
3. Hartenberg MA. Ossification centers of the pediatric elbow: a rare normal variant. Pediatr Radiol 1986; 16: 254–256.
4. Goodwin SJ, Irwin G. Normal variation in the Appearance of Elbow Ossification Centres. Brit Soc Paed Radiol annual meeting, Southampton, 2011.
5. Fowles JV, Slimane N, Kassab MT. Elbow dislocation with avulsion of the medial humeral epicondyle. J Bone Joint Surg Br 1990; 72: 102–104.
6. El-Khoury GY, Daniel WW, Kathol MH. Acute and chronic avulsive injuries. Radiol Clin North Am 1997; 35: 747–766.
7. Miles KA, Finlay DB. Disruption of the radiocapitellar line in the normal elbow. Injury 1989; 20: 365–367.
8. Donnelly LF, Klostermeier TT, Klosterman LA. Traumatic elbow effusions in pediatric patients: are occult fractures the rule? Am J Roentgenol 1998; 171: 243–245.
9. Griffith JF, Roebuck DJ, Cheng JC et al. Acute elbow trauma in children: spectrum of injury revealed by MR imaging not apparent on radiographs. Am J Roentgenol 2001; 176: 53–60.
10. Cheng JC, Ng BK, Ying SY, Lam PK. A 10 year study of the changes in the pattern and treatment of 6,493 fractures. J Pediatr Orthop 1999; 19: 344–350.
11. Rogers LF, Malave S, White H et al. Plastic bowing, torus and greenstick supracondylar fractures of the humerus; radiographic clues to obscure fractures of the elbow in children. Radiology 1978; 128: 145–150.
12. Reynolds RA, Jackson H. Concept of treatment in supracondylar humeral fractures. Injury 2005; 36: Suppl 1: S51–S56.
13. Handelsman JR. Management of fractures in children. Surg Clin North Am 1983; 63: 629–670.
14. Berman L. Personal communication, 2013.
15. Borne VD, Maaike PJ, Benjamin WL et al. The distal radioulnar joint: persisting deformity in well reduced distal radius fractures in an active population. Injury Extra 2007; 38: 377–383.

8 Adult elbow

Normal anatomy

Analysis: three questions to answer

Common injuries

A rare but important injury

Pitfalls

A child's developing skeleton is vulnerable to specific elbow injuries unlike those that affect an adult. Paediatric elbow injuries are dealt with separately in Chapter 7.

Regularly overlooked injuries

- Fracture of the radial head or neck.
- Monteggia injury[1,2].

The standard radiographs

- **AP view** in full extension.
- **Lateral** with 90° flexion.
- Routine in some departments[3]: the radial head–capitellum view (p. 121).

Abbreviations

AP, anterior-posterior; RC, radiocapitellar.

Normal Anatomy

AP view

The olecranon is obscured by the humerus. The capitellum is lateral and articulates with the radial head. The trochlea is medial and articulates with the ulna.

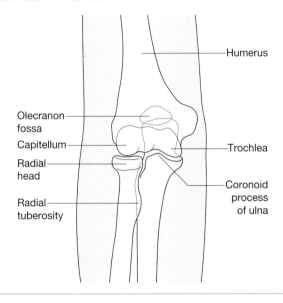

Lateral view

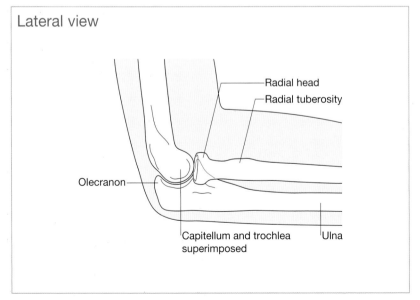

Radiocapitellar line

On the lateral view: the line to draw is along the long axis of the proximal 2–3 cm of the shaft of the radius. This line should pass through the capitellum.

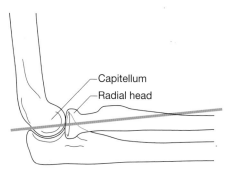

Elbow fat pads

Two pads of fat are situated close to the cortex of the distal humerus. Referred to as the anterior and posterior fat pads, these are external to the synovial lining of the joint. The fat pads are never visualised on the AP projection. Look for them on the lateral view. The fat is seen as a dark streak in the surrounding grey soft tissues.

- The anterior fat pad will be seen in most (but not all) normal elbows and is closely applied to the humerus.

- The posterior fat pad is not visible on the radiograph of a normal elbow because it is situated deep within the olecranon fossa. Because the elbow is radiographed in the flexed position this fat shadow is hidden by the overlying bone.

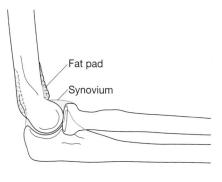

Analysis: three questions to answer

If the AP and lateral radiographs appear normal it is important that the images are again checked in a methodical manner. Ask yourself three questions.

Question 1—Are the fat pads normal on the lateral view?

The same principles apply as for the paediatric elbow (p. 102). Recap:

- Displaced anterior fat pad = possible fracture.
- Displaced posterior fat pad = probable fracture.
- Fat pads not displaced = occasionally a fracture.

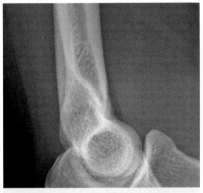

The black stripe against the anterior cortex of the humerus is a normally positioned anterior fat pad. Normal elbow.

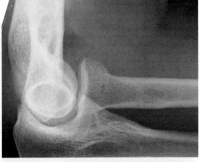

The anterior fat pad is lifted off the bone ("the sail sign") indicating an effusion. This is a variation of the standard lateral view (angled as described on p. 121). The fracture involving the head and neck of the radius is well shown.

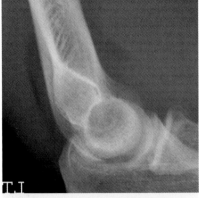

Displaced anterior and posterior fat pads. Fracture head of radius (irregularity of the anterior cortex).

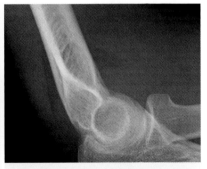

Large effusion shown by the gross displacement of the anterior and posterior fat pads. No obvious fracture on this radiograph. The AP will need careful scrutiny—particularly, the appearance of the head of the radius.

Question 2—Is the cortex of the radial head and neck smooth on both views?

- No crinkle, no step, no irregularity.
- Zoom up on the image and check that the cortex is smooth, smooth, smooth.

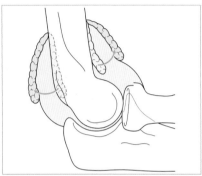

Displaced fat pads. The head of the radius shows a slight crinkle in the cortex: undisplaced fracture.

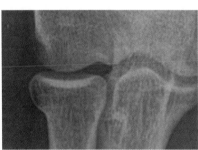

Radial head and neck. Normal cortices. No step, no crinkle, no angulation.

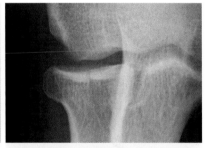

Fracture involving the head and neck of the radius. An intra-articular fracture line and a step in the lateral cortex.

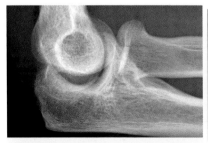

Fracture involving the head and neck of the radius. Subtle break in the articular cortex.

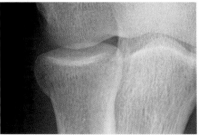

Fracture neck of radius. Subtle fracture line in the lateral cortex.

Question 3—Is the radiocapitellar (RC) line normal?[4]

Anterior dislocation of the head of radius.

The golden rule: on a normal lateral radiograph a line drawn along the long axis of the proximal 2–3 cm of the shaft of the radius should pass through the capitellum.

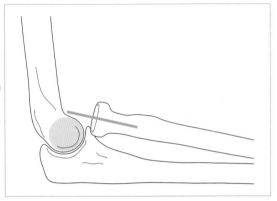

Clinical impact guideline.

Problem: Fat pad displacement but no fracture or dislocation identified after careful examination of the AP and lateral views…

Next steps:

- No additional radiographs needed. Manage as for a radial head fracture.

- Clinical review in 10 days…

  If clinically normal, no further radiography. If clinically abnormal, obtain repeat radiographs.

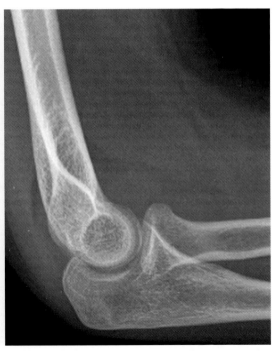

The common injuries
Fracture of the head or neck of the radius

In the adult, these fractures represent 50% of all fractures at the elbow.

An additional radiograph. Some Emergency Departments routinely add a third (an angled) projection to the standard AP and lateral views. This is termed the radial head-capitellum view[3]. The patient is positioned as for the lateral view but the tube is angled 45° to the joint. This is an excellent projection for evaluation of the radial head.

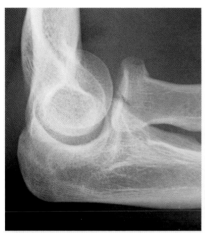

Angled projection. Fracture of radial head and neck.

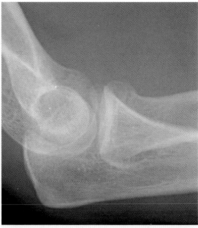

Fracture through the radial neck.

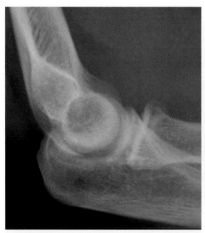

Slight kink indicates a fracture of the radial neck.

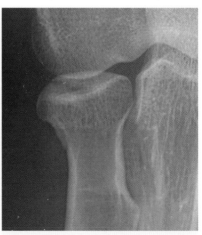

Fracture of the radial head and neck.

Fracture of the olecranon[5]

Accounts for 10-20% of adult elbow fractures.

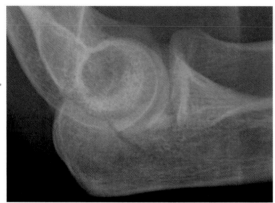

Undisplaced fracture involving the olecranon.

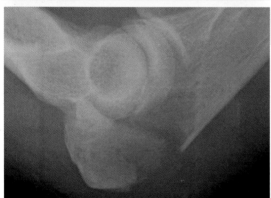

Displaced fracture of the olecranon.

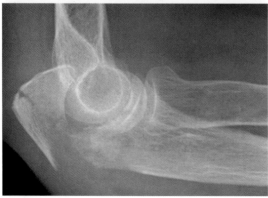

Comminuted fracture of the olecranon.

The major fragment is widely displaced posteriorly.

A rare but important injury

The Monteggia injury[1,2,5]

This combination injury represents less than 5% of all elbow fractures or dislocations[4-6]. Often referred to as a Monteggia fracture–dislocation or a Monteggia lesion. It comprises a fracture of the ulna and dislocation of the head of the radius.

Background: the forearm bones can be regarded as acting as a single functional unit as they are bound together by the strong interosseous membrane and ligaments. Consequently, a displaced or angulated fracture of just one of these two bones will be accompanied by an injury affecting the other bone—invariably a dislocation. Whenever there is a displaced fracture of the ulna, but an intact radius it is important to assess the proximal radio-ulnar joint for a dislocation of the head of the radius utilising the radiocapitellar line. This assessment will show whether a Monteggia injury is present.

Clinical impact guideline: early diagnosis is clinically very important… *"the key to a good result following a Monteggia fracture–dislocation is prompt recognition of the injury pattern"*[2].

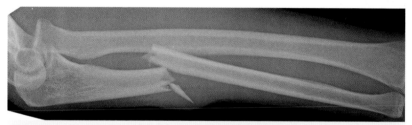

Monteggia injury. Comminuted, displaced, and angulated fracture of the ulna. Intact radius. Abnormal radiocapitellar line reveals a dislocation of the head of the radius. This injury follows the principle of the Two Bone Rule (p. 146).

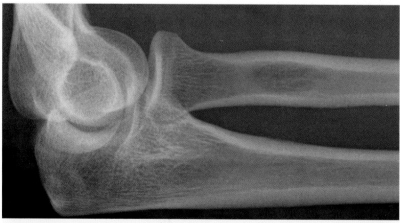

An angled projection (see p. 121) showing normal alignment of the head of the radius with the capitellum. The radiocapitellar line (p. 117) is unquestionably normal.

123

Pitfalls

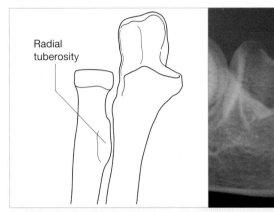

Radial tuberosity

A common normal variant. The tuberosity of the radius can cause a difficulty. The tendon of the biceps muscle is attached to this tuberosity. On the lateral view the normal tuberosity may be seen *en face* and, because of the relative density of the margins of the tuberosity, it can appear as an oval lucency. This lucency may be mistaken for an area of bone destruction or a bone cyst[6]. The apparent "cyst" in the shaft of this radius is entirely normal. Another example is evident on p. 123.

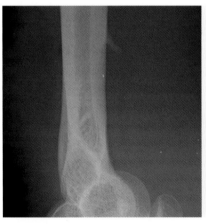

An occasional normal variant. This upper arm was lacerated by a glass bottle. The lateral radiograph showed this density anterior to the shaft of the humerus above the elbow. This is not a glass fragment. It is an atavistic supracondylar spur.

A supracondylar spur occurs in 1–2% of normal individuals. It is a normal structure in some mammals, particularly climbing animals[7]. In clinical practice it is usually an incidental and unimportant finding. Occasionally a spur may cause symptoms usually related to its effect on the median or ulnar nerve.

References

1. David-West KS, Wilson NI, Sherlock DA et al. Missed Monteggia injuries. Injury 2005; 36: 1206–1209.
2. Ring D, Jupiter JB, Simpson NS. Monteggia fractures in adults. J Bone Joint Surg 1998; 80: 1733–1744.
3. Greenspan A, Norman A. The radial head, capitellum view: useful technique in elbow trauma. Am J Roentgenol 1982; 138: 1186–1188.
4. Miles KA, Finlay DB. Disruption of the radiocapitellar line in the normal elbow. Injury 1989; 20: 365–367.
5. Rogers LF. Radiology of skeletal trauma. 3rd ed. Churchill Livingstone, 2002.
6. Keats TE, Anderson MW. Atlas of normal Roentgen variants that may simulate disease. 9th ed. Elsevier, 2012.
7. Kessel L, Rang M. Supracondylar spur of the humerus. J Bone Joint Surg 1966; 48B: 765–769.

Regularly overlooked injuries

- Undisplaced fracture of distal radius.
- Dislocation involving the lunate.
- Greenstick fracture.
- Triquetral fracture.

The standard radiographs

PA, Lateral, Scaphoid series.

Abbreviations

AVN, avascular necrosis; C, capitate; L, lunate; PA, posterior-anterior (view); R, radius.

Normal anatomy

PA projection: bones and joints

The articular surface of the radius lies distal to that of the ulna in 90% of normal people.

The carpal bones are arranged in two rows, bound together by strong ligaments:

- The joint spaces are uniform in width: 1–2 mm wide in the adult.

- Adjacent bones have parallel/congruous surfaces.

- Abnormally narrow spaces are invariably due to radiographic projection or to age related degenerative change; rarely due to injury.

- Abnormally wide spaces are likely to indicate damaged ligaments.

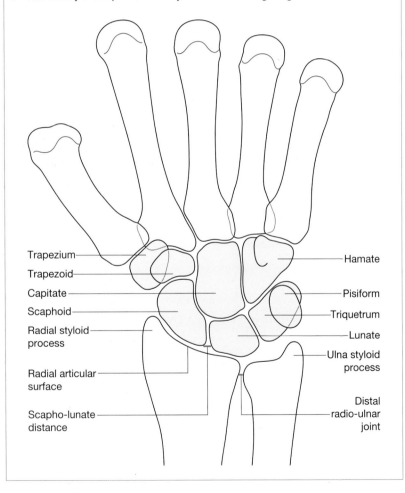

Trapezium

Trapezoid

Capitate

Scaphoid

Radial styloid process

Radial articular surface

Scapho-lunate distance

Hamate

Pisiform

Triquetrum

Lunate

Ulna styloid process

Distal radio-ulnar joint

Lateral projection: bones and joints

The dorsal cortex of the distal radius is completely smooth—no crinkles, no irregularity. This cortex should be as smooth as a baby's bottom.

The alignment of the carpal bones may appear confusing but identifying the important anatomy is actually very simple. Don't worry about the overlapping bones. Just think: apple, cup, saucer.

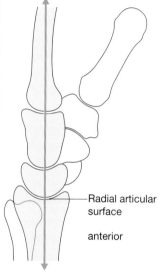

Radial articular surface

anterior

The distal radius, the lunate and the capitate articulate with each other and lie in a straight line; like an apple in a cup sitting on a saucer. The radius (R, the saucer) holds the lunate (L, the cup) and the cup of the lunate contains the capitate (C, the apple).

The articular surface of the radius has a slight but definite palmar (ie anterior) tilt. The angle of tilt is usually about 10°, but ranges from 2° to 20°.

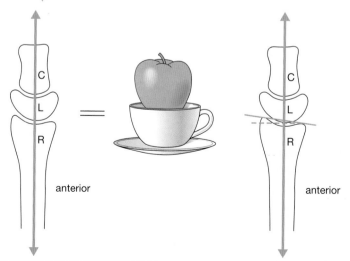

anterior

anterior

Analysis: the checklists

The PA view will appear fairly comforting to an inexperienced observer because all of the carpal bones are clearly shown. The lateral radiograph may appear terrifyingly complex and difficult to analyse because of the numerous overlapping bones. There is a very clear message: **do not be afraid!**

The lateral view is diagnostically very, very, important, so we will show you how to quickly and confidently analyse every lateral radiograph using a simple checklist.

The PA view

Analysis: ask yourself five questions.

Questions 1–4 apply to all adults. Question 5 applies to all children.

1. Is the radial articular surface and/or the ulna styloid process whole and intact?

   No = undisplaced fracture.

2. Does the radial articular surface lie distal to the ulna?

   No = suspect disruption at the radio-ulnar joint.

3. Is the scaphoid bone intact and normal?

   No = fracture.

4. Is the scapho-lunate distance less than 2 mm wide?

   No = suspect a tear of the scapho-lunate ligaments (p. 147).

5. In children: does the radial cortex show any angulation or any suggestion of a localised bulge?

   Yes = Greenstick or Torus fracture.

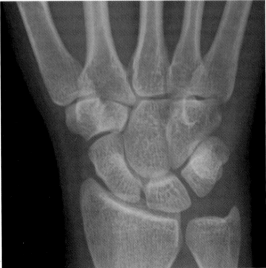

Normal PA wrist.

The answer to questions 1–4 is yes.

Abnormal PA wrist.

(1) Subtle increase in density of the metaphysis of the radius suggests an impacted fracture.

(2) Widening of the distal radio-ulnar joint and the ulnar articular surface lies distal to the immediately adjacent radial articular surface. The radio-ulnar joint is disrupted.

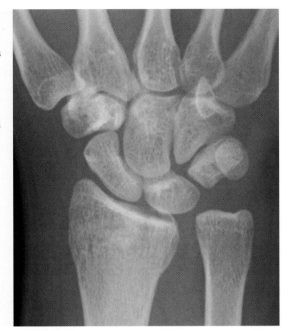

Abnormal PA wrist.

A subtle lucent line crosses the metaphyseal–diaphyseal region of the radius.

Note the slight bulging of the adjacent cortex.

Fracture of the radius. A Torus fracture (p. 18)

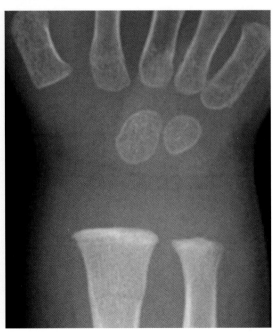

Wrist & distal forearm

The lateral view

Analysis: ask yourself five simple questions on each and every lateral view. No exceptions.

If you ask and correctly answer these five questions you will detect all the subtle and clinically important abnormalities.

1. Is the radial articular surface intact?

    No = undisplaced fracture.

2. Is the dorsal cortex of the distal radius smooth? Specifically:

    ☐   Is the cortex as smooth as a baby's bottom?

    ☐   No crinkle, no angulation, no bulge, no buckling?

    ☐   Are you sure? Check the dorsal cortex one more time.

    No, it is not smooth = undisplaced fracture.

3. Is the palmar tilt (normal range 2–20°) of the articular surface of the radius normal?

    No = suspect an impacted fracture.

4. Is there a bone fragment lying posterior to the carpal bones?

    Yes = Triquetral fracture.

5. Is there a bone sitting in the cup of the lunate?

    No = carpal dislocation involving the lunate (pp. 148–150).

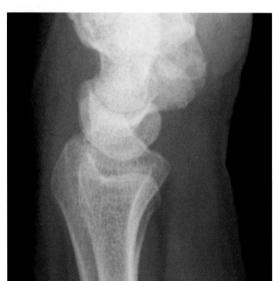

Normal lateral wrist.

Normal palmar tilt. Dorsal cortex of the radius is as smooth as a baby's bottom. The cup of the lunate is full—it articulates normally with the capitate.

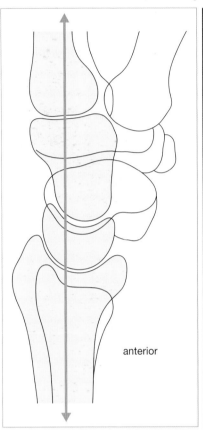

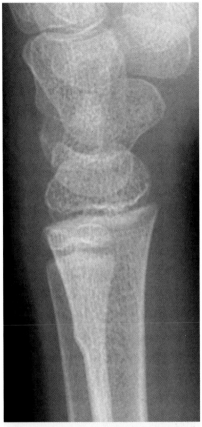

The three bones (radius, lunate, capitate) are in line. Normal appearance.

Child. Injured wrist. Slight kink and angulation in the dorsal cortex of the radial diaphysis. Greenstick fracture.

The scaphoid series

Many undisplaced scaphoid fractures are not visualised on the two standard (wrist) views. Two extra views produces a better return. Therefore, a four view scaphoid series is essential and should be requested whenever there is 'snuffbox' tenderness:

The two additional images will vary between Emergency Departments. Importantly, two of the four projections will always include a true PA and a true lateral of the wrist.

Scaphoid fractures are mainly hairline fractures and lucent; they are not sclerotic. Occasionally the fracture is displaced.

Analysis: ask yourself three questions.

1. Does the scaphoid appear intact on each of the four views?

    No = fracture (see p. 144).

2. Is the distal radius—particularly the styloid process—intact?

    No = fracture (see pp. 136–141).

    AND

3. Have I checked the PA and lateral views step-by-step (see pp. 128–130)?

    No = start checking.

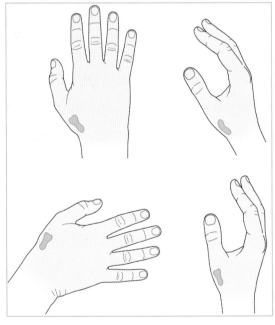

Snuffbox tenderness. A four view scaphoid series.

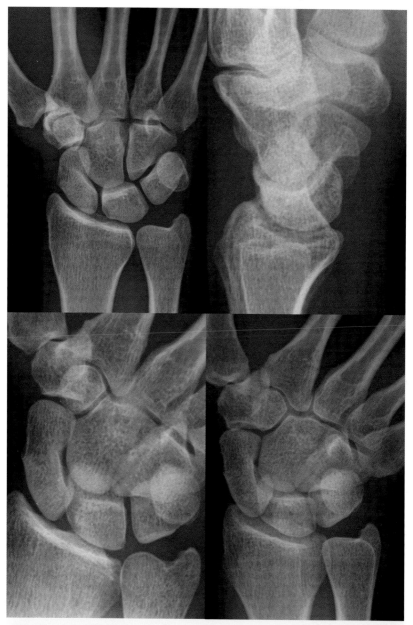

A four view scaphoid series. Normal.

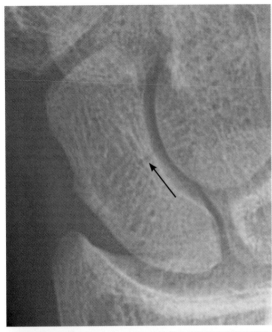

Hairline fracture (arrow) through the waist of the scaphoid.

This is the most typical appearance.

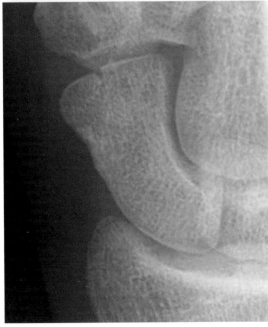

Fracture of the distal pole of the scaphoid.

Distal pole fractures are comparatively infrequent.

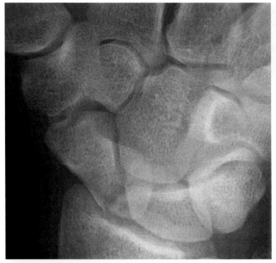

Fracture of the proximal pole of the scaphoid.

Proximal pole fractures are comparatively infrequent.

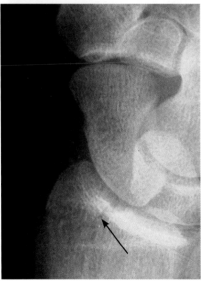

One view from a scaphoid series. The scaphoid is intact but there is an undisplaced fracture of the radial styloid (arrow). The distal radius must be evaluated very carefully on every scaphoid series—snuffbox tenderness is often due to a fracture of the radius.

Wrist myths

Inevitably there will be some soft tissue swelling over the site of an injury due to simple bruising, a ligamentous injury, a fracture, or a combination of all of these. This soft tissue swelling on the radiograph is not particularly helpful in terms of radiological diagnosis. There have been claims that the appearance of some soft tissue fat stripes around the wrist can be helpful, but this is not the case[1].

135

The common fractures

Patient age and the common fractures

Age (years)	Very young (4-10)	Older children (10-16)	Young adults (17+)	Middle age (50+)	Elderly
Usual fracture	Greenstick or Torus	Epiphyseal (Salter–Harris)	Scaphoid or Triquetal	Colles'	Colles'

Fractures of the distal radius

These injuries result from a fall on the outstretched hand.

Obvious fractures

▨ Colles' fracture—radial fracture with dorsal displacement.

▨ Smiths' fracture—radial fracture with ventral displacement.

Subtle fractures/careful diagnosis

▨ A crinkle, or any irregularity of the cortex of the dorsal aspect of the distal radius.

▨ An impacted and undisplaced fracture:

⬑ The only abnormality may be a very slight increase in the density of the radial metaphysis and/or

⬑ Loss of the normal palmar tilt of the radial articular surface (see p. 127).

▨ A longitudinal fracture:

⬑ Frequently undisplaced (see p. 139)

⬑ Barton-type fractures (see p. 138).

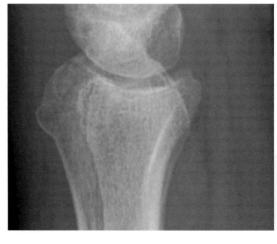

Irregular and crinkled surface of the dorsal cortex of the radius.

Undisplaced fracture.

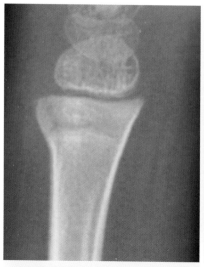

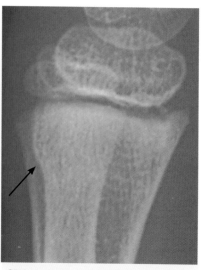

Slight angulation of the dorsal cortex of the radius. Greenstick fracture.

Slight bulge/angulation (arrow) on the dorsal cortex of the radius. A Torus (or Greenstick) fracture.

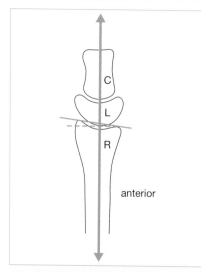

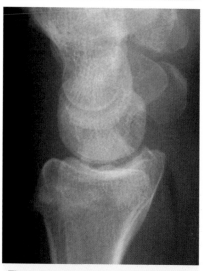

Normal. The palmar tilt of the articular surface of the radius varies between 2° and 20°. If this tilt is absent, or reversed, then an impacted fracture is probable/almost certain.

The radius shows: (1) irregularity of the dorsal cortex; (2) increase in density of the metaphysis; (3) reversal of the normal palmar tilt of the articular surface. Conclusion: impacted fracture.

137

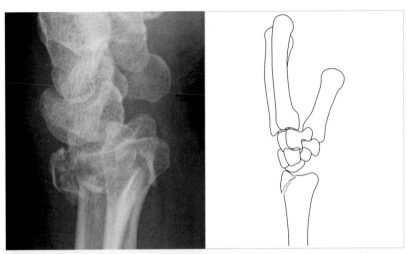

Barton fracture. A shearing fracture involving the dorsal cortex of the distal radius and its articular surface; ie it extends into the wrist joint. When the radial fragment is displaced it moves posteriorly and carries the carpus with it.

Often incorrectly assumed to be any longitudinal fracture of the distal radius.

Clinical impact guideline: Barton-type fractures are important to recognise as these are very unstable injuries. Careful evaluation of the radiographs is essential in order to make the correct diagnosis.

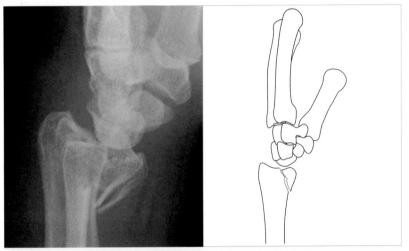

Reverse Barton fracture (volar Barton fracture). This Barton fracture variant is present when the intra-articular fracture involves the anterior cortex of the radius.

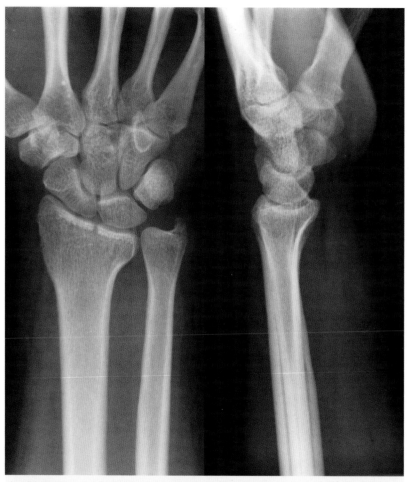

In all instances the frontal and lateral radiographs need to be evaluated as a pair. Sometimes an abnormality will be detected on the frontal view and not on the lateral radiograph, and vice versa. This patient had fallen onto an outstretched hand.

The PA view: a longitudinal fracture involving the articular surface of the radius, a fracture of the ulnar styloid process, and slight disruption of the radio-ulnar joint.

The lateral view: slight irregularity of the dorsal cortex of the distal radius. Otherwise the appearances are normal.

Principal diagnosis: undisplaced intra-articular fracture of the distal radius.

A secondary feature: subluxation at the distal radio-ulnar joint. Instability at this joint is an occasional longer term complication.

Fractures of the distal radius in children

Sometimes these fractures are obvious. Many are very subtle.

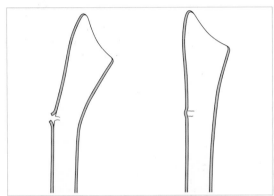

Greenstick fracture (left).

Slight angulation of the radial cortex. Note how the intact periosteum acts like a hinge.

Torus fracture (right).

Slight bulge of the radial cortex.

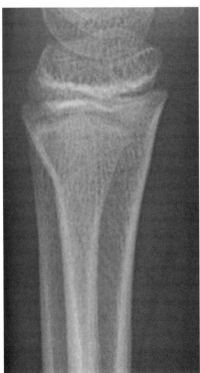

Greenstick fracture.

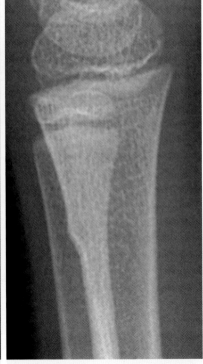

Torus fracture.

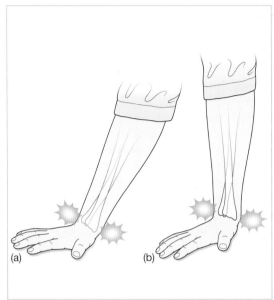

A Greenstick fracture often results from a fall with the forearm positioned at an angle to the ground (a). A Torus fracture tends to result from the forearm being in a more vertical position (b).

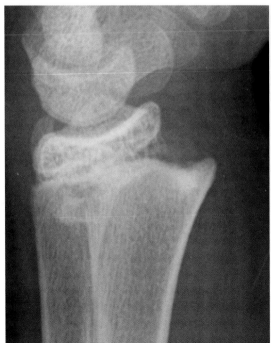

Salter–Harris fractures.

These fractures involve the growth plate. They are described in detail on pages 15–17.

This lateral radiograph shows a fracture through the growth plate of the radius. The epiphysis is displaced posteriorly. The fracture also extends into the metaphysis of the radius. This is a Salter–Harris Type 2 fracture.

Fractures of the distal ulna

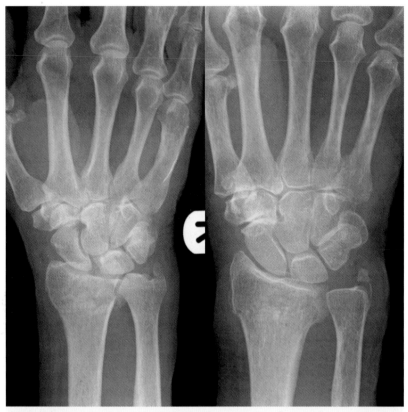

Ulna styloid fracture.

The two patients shown above had each sustained a Colles' fracture.
The lateral radiographs are not shown here.

An undisplaced fracture of the ulna styloid often accompanies a Colles' fracture, as shown above. In general, this particular ulna fracture is not itself clinically important.

However, if an ulna styloid fracture is displaced (as in the right hand image), then this can indicate that serious disruption of the distal radio-ulnar joint has occurred[2]. Consequently, instability at this joint is a possible longer term complication.

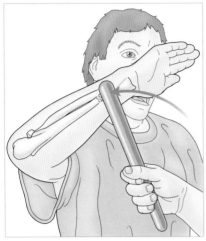

Nightstick fracture.

A Nightstick fracture is an isolated fracture of the ulna caused by a direct blow to the ulnar border of the forearm during a fight, fall, sporting activity, or car accident. Commonly, but not always, the fracture involves the middle third of the shaft of the ulna.

The term Nightstick fracture was coined because of the usual forearm defence against receiving a head injury when warding off a policeman's nightstick, or a truncheon, a crowbar, or a baseball bat. The arm is brought up above the head and consequently it is the ulna that receives the downward blow.

Clinical impact guideline: most Nightstick fractures are undisplaced or minimally displaced. However, if there is more than 50% displacement the fracture will invariably require open reduction and internal fixation.

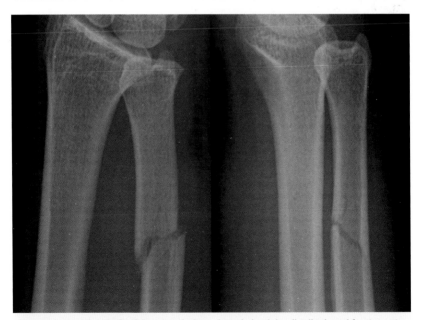

Direct blow to the shaft of the ulna during a brawl. A minimally displaced fracture at the site of the blow. A Nightstick fracture.

143

Scaphoid fracture

This injury mainly affects young adults (see p. 136). Carpal bone injuries—including scaphoid fractures—are very rare in children.

A recent scaphoid fracture is never sclerotic (ie white/dense).

Most scaphoid fractures will be evident on the initial scaphoid series[3]. Contrary to conventional teaching, the number of occult fractures revealed by repeat radiography at 10 days is very low[4,5]. Persisting clinical suspicion warrants an MRI, not more plain film radiography.

Clinical impact guideline: If a scaphoid fracture is initially overlooked and the patient is managed incorrectly then any of the following may occur: non-union, delayed union, avascular necrosis (AVN) of the proximal fragment, or osteoarthritis.

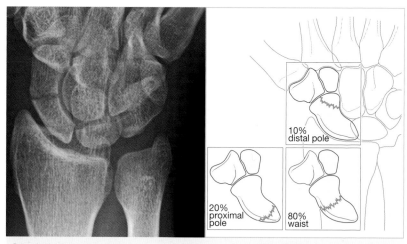

Scaphoid fracture. Fractures may involve the waist, proximal pole, or distal pole. The majority are hairline and undisplaced. A fracture across the waist jeopardises the blood supply of the proximal fragment, because the majority of the arterial supply enters via the distal pole/waist before feeding the proximal pole[6].

Risk of AVN following a scaphoid fracture

Site of fracture	Risk of AVN
Waist	High
Proximal pole	Very high
Distal pole	Nil

Triquetral fracture

A small fragment or flake of bone lying posterior to the proximal row of the carpus on the lateral view invariably represents an avulsion fracture of the triquetrum (the triquetral bone). This fracture accounts for approximately 20% of all carpal bone fractures[5].

Occasionally a triquetral fracture may occur when there is a perilunate dislocation of the carpus[6]. This emphasizes the importance of two of our basic principles:

1. Avoid a premature "satisfaction of search" approach. Complete the checklist.

2. Always check the saucer, cup, apple alignment on every lateral radiograph. Remember: the cup of the lunate should never be empty (see pp. 148–150).

Clinical impact guideline: if a solitary triquetral fracture is detected, the patient can be reassured that the injury will be treated conservatively, mainly by providing pain relief, and an excellent outcome is anticipated.

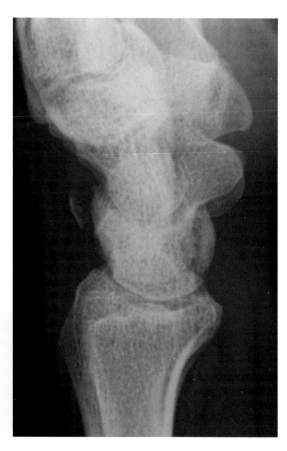

Triquetral fracture.

The small fragment of bone is an avulsed fragment from the triquetrum. The posterior position of the fragment on the lateral radiograph is typical.

Subluxations and dislocations

Distal radio-ulnar joint subluxation

Disruption of this joint is a relatively frequent finding with a Colles' fracture, occurring in 18% of cases[7]. Isolated traumatic dislocation or subluxation of this joint is rare.

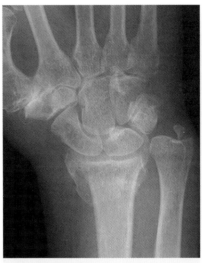

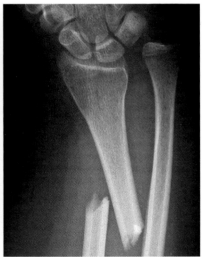

Colles' fracture. In this patient the radio-ulnar joint is also disrupted.

Radial shaft fracture. Whenever there is a fracture of the radial shaft with angulation or over-riding and an intact ulna, there will also be separation of the distal radio-ulnar joint. This combination injury is termed a Galeazzi injury. This fracture–dislocation follows the principle of the Two Bone Rule (see below).

The Two Bone Rule

In a two-bone system[8] such as the radius and ulna, where the bones are tightly bound together by an interosseous membrane and/or ligaments, the two bones can be regarded as acting as a single functional unit. In effect, they form a bound-together ring. Consequently, if only one of the bones is fractured and displaced or angulated resulting in shortening there must be a disturbance somewhere else. That disturbance may be at a joint (proximally or distally) and these joints must be carefully evaluated. Apply these guidelines when a forearm fracture is present:

- Displaced ulna fracture + normal shaft of radius
  …dislocation of the head of the radius (a Monteggia injury).

- Displaced radial fracture + normal shaft of ulna
  …distal radio-ulnar joint separation (a Galeazzi injury).

Scapho-lunate separation

The scapho-lunate joint is particularly susceptible to ligamentous injury. In adults, following an injury to the wrist, any widening of the normal space (normal = 2 mm) between the lunate and the scaphoid bones on the PA radiograph is strongly suggestive of a ligamentous tear.

This injury is particularly common in the elderly when the ligaments may be friable.

Clinical impact guidelines: The syndrome of chronic wrist pain located around the scapho-lunate joint due to scapho-lunate instability is a very troublesome problem[9]. In the elderly, this injury will usually be treated conservatively. In younger patients, surgery will be considered in order to restore full function and a pain free wrist.

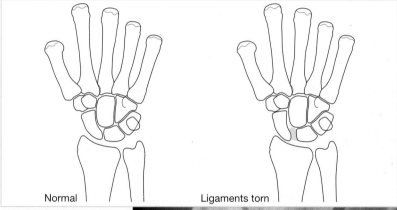

Normal   Ligaments torn

Actors and actresses rule the roost.

Terry Thomas was a 20th-century English comic actor, always grinning and showing a trademark gap between his upper incisors. Madonna, the 21st-century actress and singer, used to possess a similar dental configuration. An abnormal gap between the scaphoid and the lunate bones indicating a tear of the scapho-lunate ligaments (as shown here) is often termed the Terry Thomas or Madonna sign.

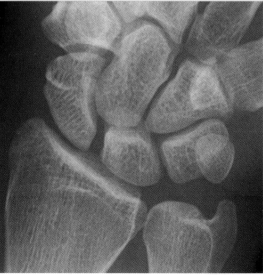

147

Rare but important injuries

Fractures of the other carpal bones

- 95% of carpal bone fractures involve the scaphoid or the triquetral bones. Fractures of the other bones do occur but are relatively uncommon.

- A fracture of the hamate may occur when a fist puncher has injured the base of his 4th or 5th metacarpal (pp. 167–168).

- The hook of the hamate may also fracture as a result of a direct blow to the carpus or as an avulsion injury associated with racquet sports or a golf swing[5,6].

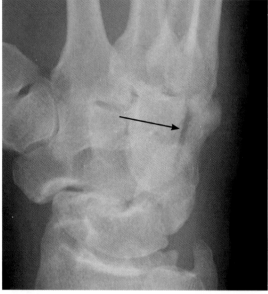

Hamate fracture (arrow).

The patient had punched a wall.

Subluxations/dislocations of the carpus

These injuries are infrequent but are usually centred around the lunate bone. The following rule is the key to their detection, and must be applied to all lateral views:

The cup of the lunate should never be empty.

Lunate dislocation and perilunate dislocations of the carpus[6,10,11]

These dislocations are not difficult to recognise provided that the basic anatomy on the lateral view is properly understood (see p. 127). The distal radius, the lunate and the capitate articulate with each other and lie in a straight line. Consequently, the question to ask on all lateral views is:

'Does a bone (the capitate) sit in the cup of the lunate?'

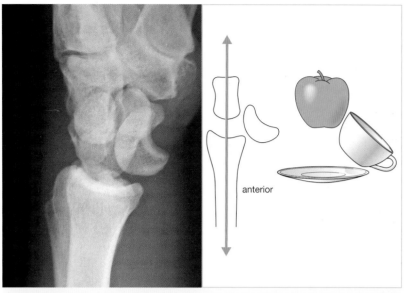

Lunate dislocation, lateral view.

The lunate dislocates anteriorly. On the lateral view the cup of the lunate is empty. The radius and the capitate remain in a straight line.

Lunate dislocation, PA view.

Emphasis is often unnecessarily placed on the appearance of the lunate on the PA view because a dislocated lunate can adopt a triangular configuration instead of its normal 'squareish' contour.

In practice, this sign is more interesting than helpful[12] because it is much easier and more definitive to diagnose a dislocation by assessing the lateral view.

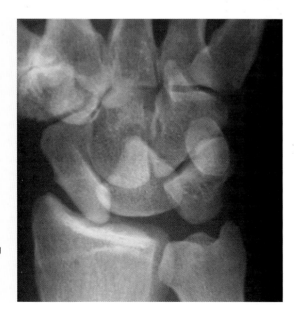

149

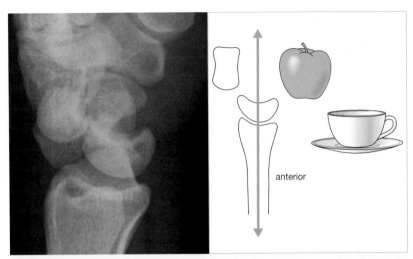

anterior

Perilunate dislocation[11]. The whole of the carpus (except for the lunate) is displaced posteriorly. Inspection of the lateral view reveals the misalignment of the carpal bones. A perilunate dislocation is often accompanied by a scaphoid fracture. Occasionally it is also associated with a triquetral fracture[6].

Satisfaction of search. Detection of a scaphoid fracture (if present) on the PA view may comfort the unwary who then fail to analyse the lateral view carefully. The unwary will overlook the following…

- The cup of the lunate is empty.

- The radius and the lunate remain in a straight line but the capitate lies posteriorly and out of line.

- In other words: the apple, the cup and the saucer do not line up. A perilunate dislocation.

Carpal subluxations[6,8]

Ligamentous tears or ruptures can affect any of the small joints of the carpus. Such injuries may result in carpal instability, pain, and reduced function.

Normally, the joint spaces between the intercarpal joints measure no more than 2 mm in the adult. Widening of any of these spaces raises the possibility of an intercarpal subluxation. In addition, subluxation will be suggested because adjacent bones do not have parallel or congruent surfaces.

Help is always available. If you are in any doubt as to whether there is true widening at a carpal joint, you can always obtain a radiograph of the uninjured wrist. This will allow comparison between the injured and uninjured sides.

Clinical impact guideline: Referral to a hand surgeon for a specialist clinical evaluation will be necessary when joint widening or lack of parallelism of adjacent surfaces is noted.

Normal variants that can mislead

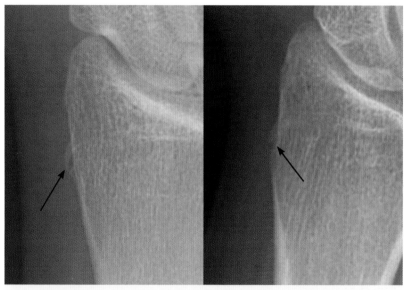

Normal radial beak. It is quite common for there to be a normal projection of bone—a beak—protruding from the lateral aspect (arrows) in the region/site of the fused growth plate.

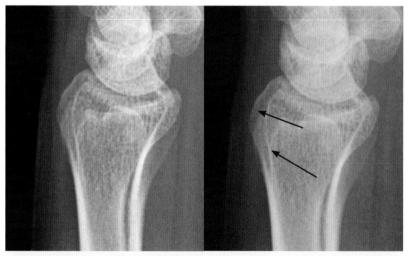

Normal longitudinal ridges. In most mature skeletons the dorsal cortex of the distal radius is a single smooth line. However, it is a common normal variant for the dorsal cortex to contain/be seen as two or three smooth longitudinal ridges (arrows).

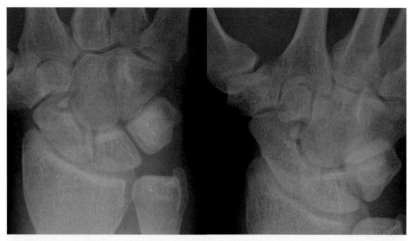

Accessory ossicles.

Several accessory carpal bones do occur; all are rare. One accessory ossicle, the os centrale carpi, can be confused with an avulsed fragment from the scaphoid bone. Its location (above) projected adjacent to the medial aspect of the distal pole of the scaphoid is typical.

References

1. Annamalai G, Raby N. Scaphoid and pronator fat stripes are unreliable soft tissue signs in the detection of radiographically occult fractures. Clin Radiol 2003; 58: 798–800.
2. McRae R, Esser M. Practical Fracture Treatment. 5th ed. Churchill Livingstone, 2008.
3. Brondum V, Larsen CF, Skov O. Fracture of the carpal scaphoid: frequency and distribution in a well defined population. Eur J Radiol 1992; 15: 118–122.
4. Low G, Raby N. Can follow-up radiography for acute scaphoid fracture still be considered a valid investigation? Clin Radiology 2005; 60: 1106–1110.
5. Raby N. Imaging of wrist trauma. In Davies AM, Grainger AJ, James SJ. Imaging of the Hand and Wrist. Springer Verlag, 2013.
6. Goldfarb CA, Yin Y, Gilula LA et al. Wrist fractures: what the clinician wants to know. Radiology 2001; 219: 11–28.
7. Malik AK, Pettit P, Compson J. Distal radioulnar joint dislocation in association with elbow injuries. Injury 2005; 36: 324–329.
8. Maaike PJ, van't Hof BW, Prins HJ et al. The distal radioulnar joint: persisting deformity in well reduced distal radius fractures in an active population. Injury Extra 2007; 38: 377–383.
9. Mayfield JK. Mechanism of carpal injuries. Clin Orthop Relat Res 1980; 149: 45–54.
10. Panting AL, Lamb DW, Noble J et al. Dislocations of the lunate with and without fracture of the scaphoid. J Bone Joint Surg Br 1984; 66B: 391–395.
11. Herzberg TJ, Comtet JJ, Linscheid RL et al. Perilunate dislocations and fracture-dislocations: a multicenter study. J Hand Surg Am 1993; 18A: 768–779.
12. The Wrist. Chan O (ed). ABC of Emergency Radiology. 3rd ed. Wiley Blackwell, 2013.

10 Hand & fingers

The standard radiographs

Depends on site of injury:

- Injury to a metacarpal or several phalanges:
  PA of hand and **oblique of entire hand and wrist**.

- Injury to the thumb or to a single digit: **PA and lateral of the digit**.

Regularly overlooked injuries

- Dislocations at 4th & 5th CMC joints.

- Fractures at base of 4th or 5th MCs.

- Fracture of the hamate.

Abbreviations

CMC, carpometacarpal;
IPJ, interphalangeal joint;
MC, metacarpal;
MCPJ, metacarpophalangeal joint;
PA, posterior-anterior (view).

Normal anatomy

Knowledge of the anatomical attachments of (a few) tendons and ligaments is essential. A seemingly trivial fragment of bone on the radiograph may indicate that a particular tendon or ligament is no longer anchored to the bone. Failure to recognise the functional implication can lead to inappropriate management.

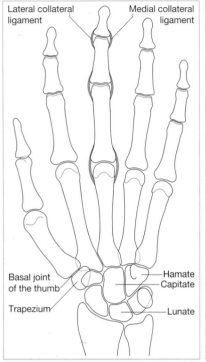

Lateral collateral ligament

Medial collateral ligament

Basal joint of the thumb

Trapezium

Hamate
Capitate

Lunate

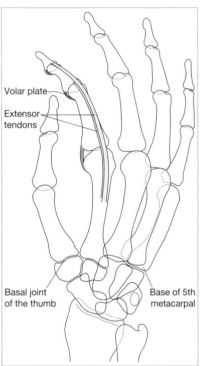

Volar plate

Extensor tendons

Basal joint of the thumb

Base of 5th metacarpal

PA view of hand and wrist.

The collateral ligaments arise from the lateral and medial margins of each metacarpal and each phalanx. They extend across the joint and insert into the same margin at the base of the adjacent phalanx.

Oblique view of hand and wrist.

The extensor tendons insert into the dorsal surface at the base of each phalanx.

The volar plate is a fibrous thickening of the joint capsule on the palmar aspect of each joint. It is attached to the bases of the adjacent phalanges.

154

The thumb

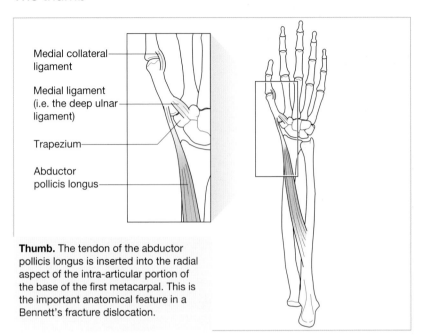

Medial collateral ligament

Medial ligament (i.e. the deep ulnar ligament)

Trapezium

Abductor pollicis longus

Thumb. The tendon of the abductor pollicis longus is inserted into the radial aspect of the intra-articular portion of the base of the first metacarpal. This is the important anatomical feature in a Bennett's fracture dislocation.

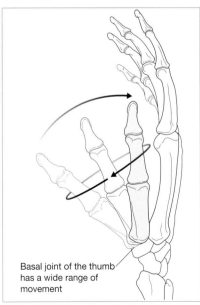

Basal joint of the thumb has a wide range of movement

Thumb.

The stability of the carpometacarpal (CMC) joint of the thumb depends on fairly lax but very tough capsular ligaments[1]. The deep ulnar ligament is the thickened part of the capsule on the palmar aspect of the 1st CMC joint. This strong ligament extends from the first metacarpal to the trapezium. The capsular ligaments and the shape of the first CMC joint (ie the trapezium–metacarpal joint) enables the thumb to adopt an extraordinary degree of mobility including the crucial ability of opposition.

1st CMC joint = basal joint of the thumb.

155

Hand & fingers

The carpometacarpal (CMC) joints

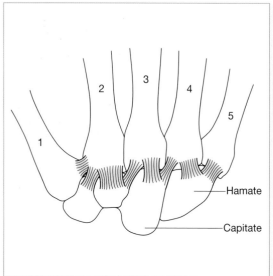

The 2nd and 3rd metacarpals are attached to the distal row of the carpal bones by thick, strong, ligaments.

The 4th and 5th metacarpals have fewer ligaments anchoring them[2]. These two CMC joints are consequently: (a) very mobile, and (b) vulnerable to injury.

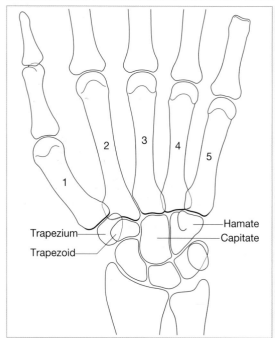

On the PA view of the hand:

- The articular cortex at the base of each metacarpal parallels the articular surface of the adjacent carpal bone.

- The CMC joint spaces are clearly seen; they are equal (approximately 1–2 mm) in width.

- The 2nd to 5th CMC joints are visualised as a zigzag tram line[3] (see opposite).

The normal CMC joints

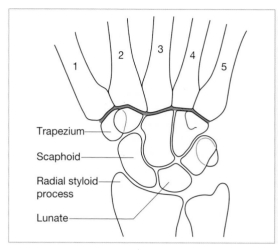

1
2
3
4
5

Trapezium

Scaphoid

Radial styloid process

Lunate

On the PA radiograph, the joint surfaces of the 2nd through to the 5th metacarpal and their adjacent carpal bones articulate, and their articular surfaces parallel one another. These joints are thus seen as a zigzag tram line[3], shown as a thick dark line on this drawing.

The zigzag line is analogous to "seeing the light of day" through each of the CMC joints.

Useful rule:

On a normal PA view of the hand there will always—yes, always—be "the light of day" seen between the bases of the 4th and 5th metacarpals and the hamate bone.

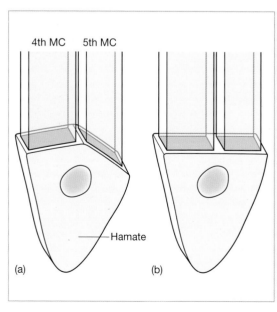

4th MC   5th MC

Hamate

(a)   (b)

A stylised drawing of the important alignment between the bases of the hamate and the 4th and 5th CMC joints. Understanding the radiographic appearance of these two joints on the PA view is important. In some people the normal joints look like (a); in others the normal joints look more like (b).

See also pp. 167–168.

Analysis: the checklist

Adopt a three-step approach:

1. Target the precise clinical site of injury.

2. Search for fractures and for any evidence of subluxation/dislocation.

3. Review the relevant muscle and ligamentous attachments because a small fracture may indicate a big loss of function.

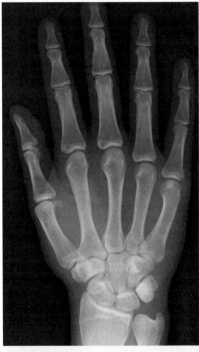

Hand, PA view.

Check for fractures, dislocations, and subluxations; check whether the 4th and 5th carpometacarpal (CMC) joints show "the light of day" (p. 157); check the basal joint of the thumb; if there is a fracture of the 1st metacarpal determine whether it is intra-articular (Bennett's fracture) or extra-articular. This is a normal PA view.

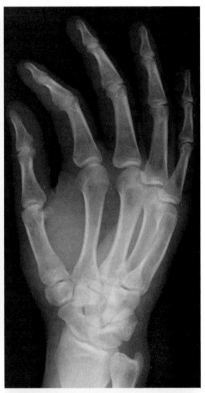

Hand, oblique view.

Check for fractures, dislocations and subluxations. This, the routine second view, will invariably clarify/categorise any abnormality that is suspected on the PA radiograph. This is a normal oblique view.

**Injury to the basal joint
of the thumb.**

An intra-articular fracture
of the base of the 1st
metacarpal.

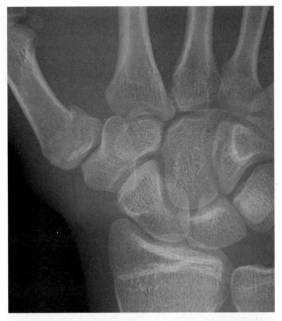

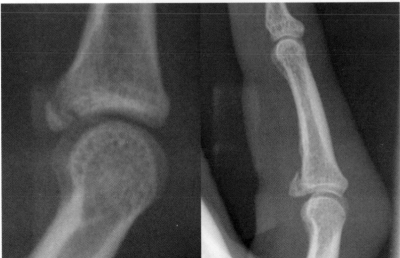

Single digit injury.

Check for fracture and dislocation/subluxation. These two patients have sustained
a volar plate injury (ie a fragment is detached from the capsular region of the palmar
aspect of an interphalangeal joint).

The common injuries

Fractures of the phalanges or metacarpals

Most fractures involving the mid-shaft of a phalanx or metacarpal are stable and pose few clinical problems. Phalangeal fractures are frequently managed by strapping to an adjacent digit (ie garter strapping or buddy strapping).

There are some "problem fractures", for which careful orthopaedic assessment is essential. The most common of these are shown on the next four pages.

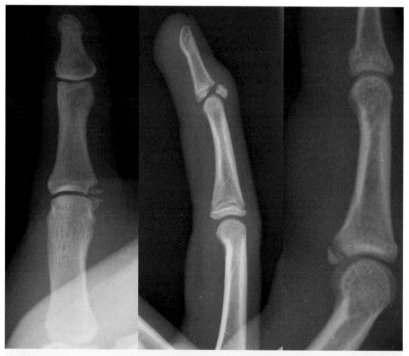

Avulsion of a small fragment at the base of a phalanx.

The ligament or tendon most likely to be compromised is indicated by the position of the fragment:

- A lateral or medial fragment indicates avulsion of the collateral ligament (left)

- A dorsal fragment indicates avulsion of the extensor tendon (middle)

- A palmar fragment indicates an avulsion of the volar plate.

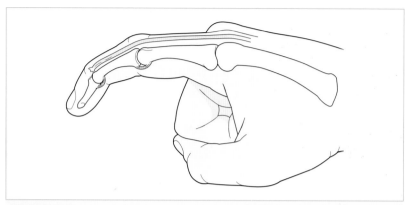

Mallet finger.

A flexion deformity (known as a mallet or baseball finger) of the distal phalanx.

An isolated flexion deformity is almost impossible without either a rupture of the extensor tendon or an avulsion fracture.

A deformity necessitates very careful clinical examination because a fracture is present in only 25% of mallet fingers.

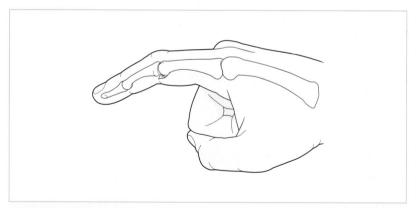

Volar plate fracture.

Caused by forced extension of a finger.

The detached fragment will be visualised on the oblique view—not on the PA view.

These fractures are nearly always displaced and thus unstable.

161

Spiral fracture of the shaft of a phalanx or metacarpal.

These fractures are often unstable and significant shortening may occur. The fracture frequently requires open reduction and internal fixation[4].

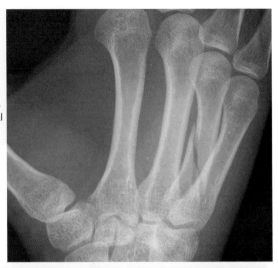

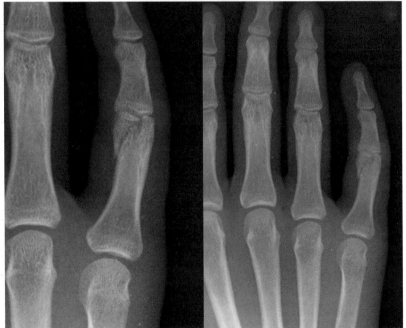

Fracture involving a joint surface.

If there is displacement and/or comminution then surgical repair can be challenging because the fragments are invariably very small[5].

Fracture of a metacarpal neck: Boxer's fracture.

"Boxer's fracture" is the accepted generic term when referring to a fracture of the neck of a metacarpal—frequently the 4th or 5th metacarpal. Invariably, the fracture is consequent on punching a solid object whilst the fist is clenched. The solid object might be a wall or a goal post (frustration/temper) or a chin (brawling/fist fight).

Nomenclature. The term Boxer's fracture is arguably a misnomer because trained boxers rarely fracture these particular metacarpals. Indeed, it is the untrained street fighter and not a boxer who usually presents with this injury. Background:

- A trained boxer's fracture: in the boxing ring, the athlete strikes with the wrist in the neutral position. The result is an occasional fracture of the 2nd or 3rd metacarpal, but rarely a fracture of the 4th or 5th metacarpal.

- A street fighter's (or scrapper's) fracture: when the blow is struck, the wrist is flexed. The result is a fracture of the 4th or 5th metacarpal.

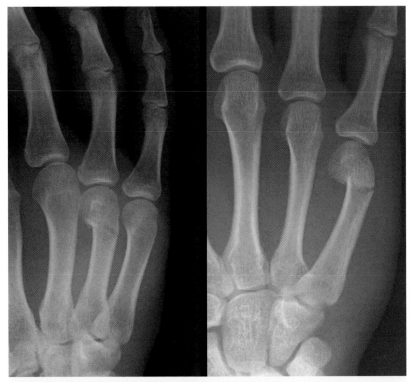

Boxer's fracture. These two patients have sustained a fracture through the neck of a metacarpal (left, 4th metacarpal; right, 5th metacarpal).

Uncommon but important injuries

Fractures and dislocations involving the thumb

The basal joint (ie the carpometacarpal or CMC joint) of the thumb is remarkable. It is multifunctional. It can adduct, abduct, oppose and circumduct (see p. 155). If the multifunctional ability of this joint is to be maintained then any injury close to this joint needs to be recognised, characterized, and treated early[1,6].

Distinguishing between an intra-articular and an extra-articular fracture at the base of the thumb is crucial. The distinction determines the appropriate treatment.

Base of thumb: extra-articular fracture

The fracture line is distal to the joint capsule. Consequently it is distal to both the deep ulnar ligament and to the insertion of the tendon of abductor pollicis longus and there is no involvement of the CMC joint and no risk of dislocation.

This is important because almost all extra-articular fractures at the base of the thumb are treated simply by closed reduction.

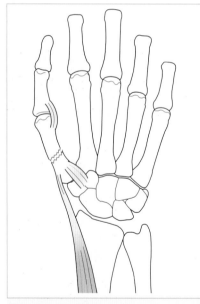

Base of thumb fracture.

The fracture line is distal to the insertion of the tendon of the abductor pollicis longus muscle. The CMC joint is not involved.

No risk of dislocation.

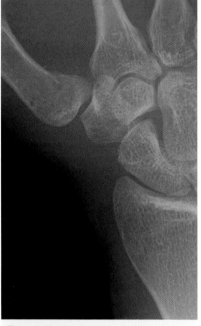

Extra articular fracture, base of 1st metacarpal.

The articular surface is not involved. The proximal fragment remains in a stable position.

Base of thumb: intra-articular fracture

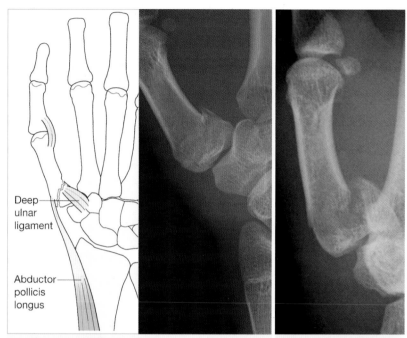

Deep ulnar ligament

Abductor pollicis longus

Bennett's fracture.

A fracture involving the base of the 1st metacarpal. Crucially, the joint surface is involved.

The larger metacarpal fragment is pulled dorsally and radially by the abductor pollicis longus muscle.

This injury is more properly termed a Bennett's fracture–dislocation. It is unstable.

Early orthopaedic treatment (often open reduction) is essential because retention of the multiple movements at this special CMC joint are so important[4,6].

Rolando's fracture.

A comminuted intra-articular fracture of the base of the 1st metacarpal. The comminuted fragments often adopt a Y, V or T configuration. It is highly unstable.

This fracture can be difficult to treat because of the comminution and displacement of the articular fragments.

Gamekeeper's/Skier's thumb[7]

■ Rupture or severe stretching of the ulnar collateral ligament (p. 155) at the first metacarpophalangeal joint (MCPJ). Occasionally a bone fragment may be avulsed. A complete tear of the ligament requires surgical repair[7,8].

  ❏ Usually the ligament alone is torn and the radiographs appear normal.

  ❏ If there is clinical uncertainty as to whether the ligament is torn then stress radiographs can assist in confirming or excluding the diagnosis. Diagnostic ultrasound examination by a skilled practitioner is a reliable alternative to stress radiography[7,8].

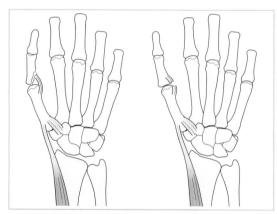

Skier's thumb.

In most cases the medial collateral ligament is torn and the standard radiographs appear normal.

Occasionally there is an avulsion fracture of the base of the proximal phalanx at the insertion of the ligament.

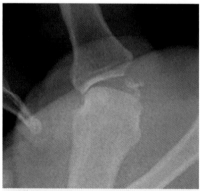

Skier's thumb.

Fragments have been detached from the base of the proximal phalanx of the thumb. This represents an avulsion (rather than a tear or stretching) of the medial collateral ligament. Result: an unstable joint.

Killing rabbits versus a Skiing wipeout

Gamekeeper's thumb results from the *chronic stretching* of the ulnar collateral ligament. So called because of the method employed by 18th and 19th century English gamekeepers to dispatch and break the necks of numerous rabbits.

Skier's thumb can occur on the ski slope when the thumb is caught against the handle of a ski pole during a fall or a wipeout. This causes an *acute tear* of the ulnar collateral ligament. A Skier's thumb comprises 15–20% of downhill skiing injuries[9]. In some countries without snow, the most common cause for a skier's thumb injury is a simple fall or a non-skiing sports injury.

Carpometacarpal (CMC) joint dislocations[3, 10–14]

High velocity motor vehicle trauma can cause a dislocation at any of the CMC joints. In less violent impacts (eg punching a wall) it is the 4th and 5th metacarpals that are most commonly dislocated.

4th or 5th CMC dislocation

Emergency Departments that receive hand injuries due to fist fights will regularly see dislocations involving these CMC joints. The injury commonly results from a transmitted force along the metacarpal shaft when the closed fist hits a solid object. It is often associated with a fracture at the base of the affected metacarpal and/or the adjacent metacarpal and/or the hamate. A fracture of the dorsal surface of the hamate (seen on the oblique view) should always raise the suspicion of a dislocation at the 5th CMC joint.

What to look for on the PA radiograph:

▨ Effacement of the adjacent CMC joint space.

▨ Apply this analogy: can I see "the light of day" (pp. 156–157) between the bases of the 4th and 5th metacarpals and the hamate? In other words, any lack of parallelism between the base of a metacarpal and the articular surface of the adjacent carpal bone (p. 168) is very suggestive of a dislocation.

▨ Has the head of the 5th metacarpal dropped well below the 4th metacarpal head?

How to confirm/refute your suspicion:

▨ Check the oblique radiograph. Then, if there is still continuing doubt, obtain a lateral view. The base of the 5th metacarpal dislocates posteriorly.

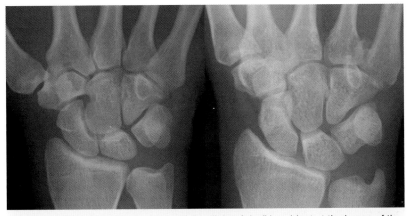

The PA image on the left is normal and the "light of day" is evident at the bases of the 4th and 5th metacarpals. The PA image on the right shows (a) fracture of the base of the 5th metacarpal and (b) loss of the joint space at the 5th CMC joint (ie indicating a dislocation). Note that the joint space ("the light of day") is well seen at the base of the 4th metacarpal indicating that this joint is normal.

The 4th and 5th CMC joints on the PA radiograph

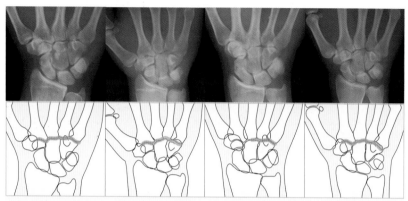

Four different patients, each with a normal PA radiograph. The corresponding artworks show that the normal carpometacarpal (CMC) joints can vary slightly in appearance between patients. The difference is invariably due to the different slope of the articular surfaces between normal patients, as illustrated in (a) and (b) below. However, when you inspect the PA view a joint space (ie a black line) at the base of the 4th and 5th metacarpals will always be visible on a normal PA radiograph, without exception. Visualising this normal zigzag black line may be conceptually difficult for an inexperienced observer. The schematic drawings below explain how a joint ("the light of day") disappears on the PA view when a 4th or 5th CMC joint is dislocated.

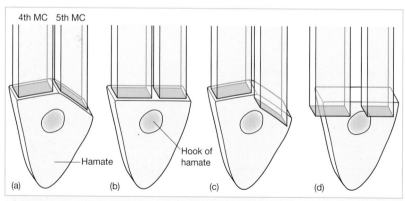

Diagrammatic representation of the 4th and 5th CMC joints.
(a) = normal; (b) = normal; (c) = dislocated 5th CMC joint;
(d) = Dislocations at 4th and 5th CMC joints.

Pitfalls

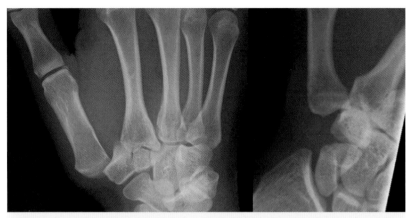

Mobile basal joint of the thumb. The exceptional mobility of the basal joint (ie the trapezium–1st metacarpal joint) of the thumb means that it may be entirely normal (above) but appears to be subluxed. Be careful not to make this mistake. Clinical correlation should discount this possibility.

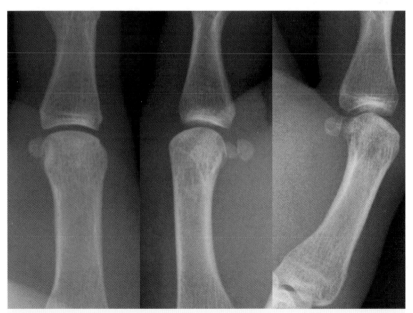

Additional bones. Sesamoid bones adjacent to the first metacarpophalangeal joint (MCPJ) should not be confused with fracture fragments. Most hands usually have five sesamoid bones: two adjacent to the MCPJ of the thumb, one adjacent to the MCPJ of the index finger and one adjacent to the MCPJ of the little finger.

Accessory epiphyses

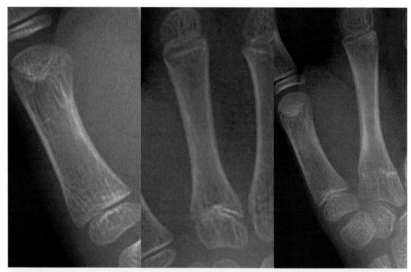

Sometimes accessory metacarpal epiphyses—or partial epiphyses—are present in young children. The most common of these *pseudoepiphyses* occur in the head of the 1st (thumb) metacarpal (left and right) and at the base of the 2nd metacarpal (centre and right). Unless the possibility of an accessory epiphysis is considered, particularly at the base of the 2nd metacarpal, then a normal developmental variant may be read as an undisplaced metacarpal fracture.

References

1. Kauer JM. Functional anatomy of the carpometacarpal joint of the thumb. Clin Orthop Relat Res 1987; 220: 7–13.
2. Mueller JJ. Carpometacarpal dislocations: report of five cases and review of the literature. J Hand Surg Am 1986; 11: 184–188.
3. Fisher MR, Rogers LF, Hendrix RW. Systematic approach to identifying fourth and fifth carpometacarpal joint dislocations. Am J Roentgenol 1983; 140: 319–324.
4. Buchholz RW, Hickman JD, Court-Brown C (eds). Rockwood and Green's Fractures in Adults. 6th ed. Lippincott Williams & Wilkins, 2006; 1211–1255.
5. Khan W, Fahmy N. The S-Quattro in the management of sports injuries of the fingers. Injury 2006; 37: 860–868.
6. Howard FM. Fractures of the basal joint of the thumb. Clin Orthop Relat Res 1987; 220: 46–51.
7. Chuter GS, Muwanga CL, Irwin LR. Ulnar collateral ligament injuries of the thumb: 10 years of surgical experience. Injury 2009; 40: 652–656.
8. Ebrahim FS, De Maeseneer M, Jager T et al. US diagnosis of UCL tears of the thumb and Stener lesions: technique, pattern-based approach, and differential diagnosis. Radiographics 2006; 26 (4): 1007–1020.
9. Engkvist O, Balkfors B, Lindsjo U. Thumb injuries in downhill skiing. Int J Sports Med 1982; 3: 50–55.
10. Gilula LA. Carpal injuries: analytic approach and case exercises. Am J Roentgenol 1979; 133: 503–517.
11. Pope TL, Harris JH (eds). Harris & Harris' The Radiology of Emergency Medicine. 5th ed. Lippincott Williams & Wilkins, 2012.
12. Rogers LF. Radiology of Skeletal Trauma. 3rd ed. Churchill Livingstone, 2002.
13. Raby N. Imaging of wrist trauma. In Davies AM, Grainger AJ, James SJ. Imaging of the Hand and Wrist. Springer Verlag, 2013.
14. Henderson JJ, Arafa MA. Carpometacarpal dislocation. An easily missed diagnosis. J Bone Joint Surg Br 1987; 69: 212–214.

11 Cervical spine

Regularly overlooked injuries

The most common causes of a missed C-spine abnormality are failure to adequately visualise the injured region and inadequate understanding of the C1/C2 anatomy. Therefore errors commonly relate to:

- C1/C2 fractures or subluxations.
- Low C-spine fractures[1–4], frequently involving the C7 vertebra.

The standard radiographs

Three-view trauma series.

Abbreviations

AP, anterior-posterior projection;
C-spine, cervical spine;
C1, Atlas vertebra;
C2, Axis vertebra;
CT, computed tomography;
ED, Emergency Room/Department;
Peg, odontoid peg;
T1, first thoracic vertebra.

Cervical spine

Normal anatomy

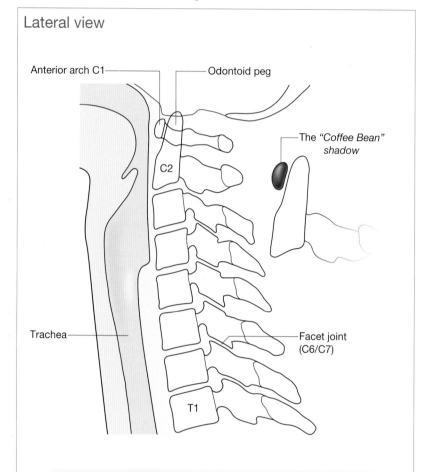

Lateral view

Anterior arch C1

Odontoid peg

The *"Coffee Bean"* shadow

C2

Trachea

Facet joint (C6/C7)

T1

The Coffee Bean Shadow.

The anterior arch of C1 is a shadow that is always visible on a lateral radiograph. It looks like a reversed capital D. We call this shadow the "Coffee Bean" shadow because we think it resembles a coffee bean. Use it as your anatomical starting point when assessing the C1–C2 anatomy.

AP Peg view

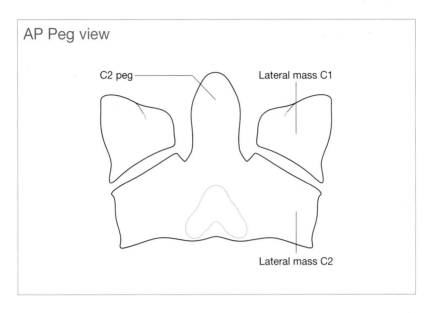

C2 peg

Lateral mass C1

Lateral mass C2

Long AP view

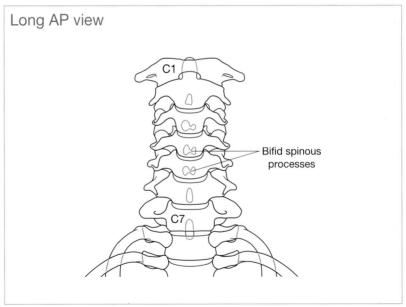

C1

Bifid spinous processes

C7

Analysis: the checklists

Injuries are most often missed because of poor radiographic technique and/ or inaccurate film interpretation[1,2,4–6]. Most errors are avoidable[5]. Missed C-spine abnormalities occur most commonly at the top or at the bottom of the C-spine[1,2].

- ❑ Whatever the level of violence, C-spine injuries frequently occur at the C1–C2 level[1,3,4,6].

- ❑ The most common fracture in elderly patients following a fall is a high cervical injury[1,3].

- ❑ Between 9% and 26% of patients with one fracture or dislocation of the spine will have further fractures demonstrable radiographically at other levels[5].

- ❑ If you have detected one injury you must still complete the checklists, in order to find any additional abnormalities.

Priority 1: Lateral view checklist

Identify the odontoid peg and assess its position and anatomical relationship to the C1 vertebra. Overlapping structures (eg mastoid, ear lobes, C1 vertebra) can make this difficult. Questions 1–5 will help you to overcome this.

Ask yourself ten important questions:

1. Is the radiograph technically adequate? Ensure that the C1–C2 articulation *and* the superior surface of the T1 vertebra are clearly seen.

2. Have I identified the anterior arch of the C1 vertebra (the "coffee bean")?

3. Is the anterior cortex of the odontoid peg (the Peg) closely apposed to the "coffee bean"?

4. Is the line of the anterior cortex of the Peg continuous with the anterior cortex of the body of C2? Any displacement implies a Peg fracture or fracture of C2 body.

5. Is the line of the posterior cortex of the Peg continuous with the posterior cortex of the body of C2? Any displacement or break indicates a Peg fracture.

6. Is Harris' ring[7] normal? A break in either the anterior or posterior margin of the ring indicates the high probability of a fracture of the Peg/body of C2 (p. 176).

7. Are the posterior arches of C1 and C2 intact?

8. Are the other vertebrae (C3–C7) intact (p. 192)?

9. Are the three main contour lines/arcs normal (p. 178)?

10. Are the pre-vertebral soft tissues normal (p. 179)?

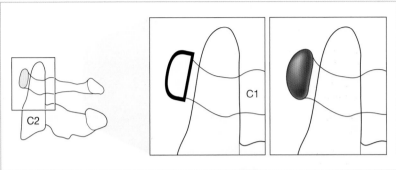

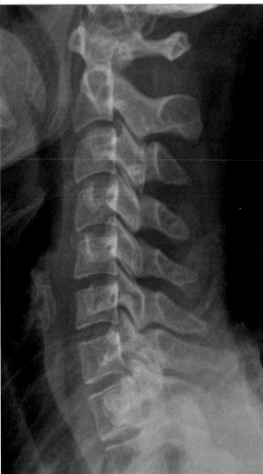

Questions 2 and 3.

Recognising the anterior arch of C1 is key to detecting the abnormalities that may involve the C2 vertebra.

The arch looks like a small coffee bean, and is always easy to identify on the lateral view.

The gap between the Peg and the coffee bean should not exceed 3 mm in adults or 5 mm in children[1].

This is a normal lateral view.

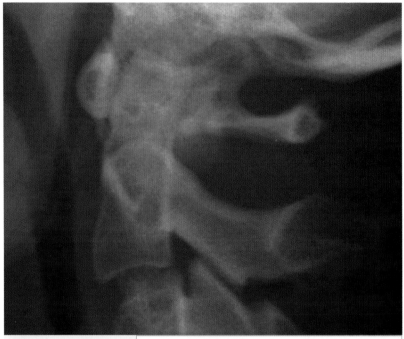

Questions 4 and 5.

Check that the anterior cortex of the Peg is continuous with the anterior cortex of the body of C2.

Also check that the posterior cortex of the Peg is continuous with the posterior cortex of the body of C2. Any displacement or break in either of these lines indicates a Peg fracture.

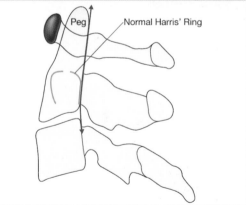

Question 6. Harris' Ring[7]. Many lateral views will show a white ring projected over the base of the Peg and over part of the body of C2 (see above). This ring may appear slightly incomplete at its inferior and/or superior aspects—that is a normal appearance. However, if either the anterior or posterior margin of the ring appears disrupted then a fracture through the base of the Peg or the body of C2 is very possible and a C2 fracture will need to be excluded (p. 188).

Question 7. Check that the posterior arches of C1 and C2 are intact.

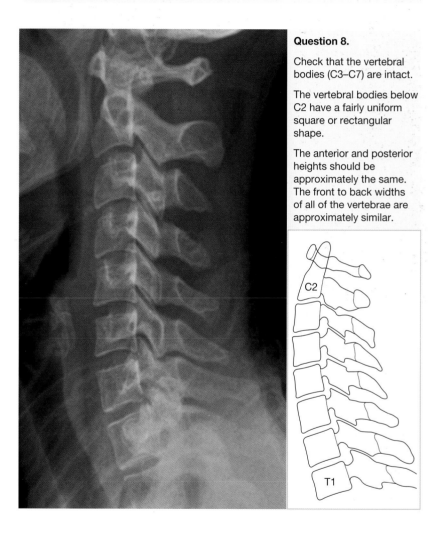

Question 8.

Check that the vertebral bodies (C3–C7) are intact.

The vertebral bodies below C2 have a fairly uniform square or rectangular shape.

The anterior and posterior heights should be approximately the same. The front to back widths of all of the vertebrae are approximately similar.

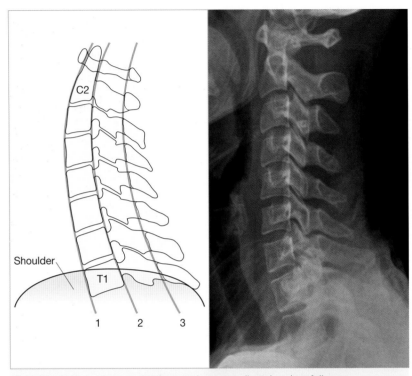

Question 9. You can trace the three main contour lines (arcs) as follows:

Line 1: along the anterior margins of the vertebral bodies (anterior line).

Line 2: along the posterior margins of the vertebral bodies (posterior line).

Line 3: along the bases of the spinous processes (spinolaminar line).

Each line should be a smooth unbroken curve or arc. No kink. No step. Trace these lines along the full length of the cervical spine. Line 1 extends from the top of the anterior cortex of the Peg to the anterior margin of the body of T1 vertebra.

Potential Pitfall: Line 3 will sometimes show a slight step at the C2 level, particularly in children[8].

Apply this rule: this step should not be more than 2 mm posterior to the smooth arc as it is traced upwards between C3 and C1 vertebrae.

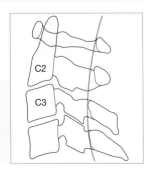

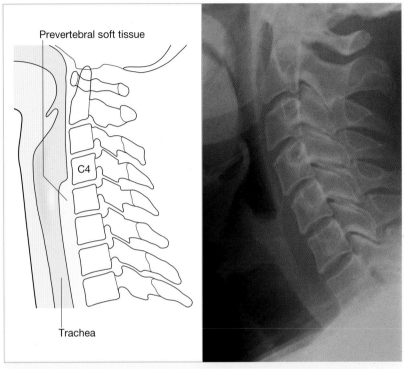

Prevertebral soft tissue

C4

Trachea

Question 10. Are the pre-vertebral soft tissue shadows normal? The soft tissue shadow[7,9–11] anterior to the vertebral bodies has a characteristic configuration and width. Any bulge or local increase in width indicates haemorrhage and connotes an important injury.

NB: The absence of a bulge does not exclude a ligamentous or bone injury. Indeed, even with a major injury, a soft tissue bulge due to a haematoma is fairly rare.

Maximum normal width of the prevertebral soft tissues

Level	Width	Approximate % of a vertebral body (AP) width
C1–C4	7 mm	30%
C5–C7	22 mm	100%

Cervical spine

Priority 2: AP Peg view checklist

The anatomical arrangement of the C1–C2 articulation allows extensive neck rotation whilst providing maximum stability. This stability depends on the integrity of the ligaments, particularly the C2 transverse ligament. Various other ligaments enable C1 vertebra to be held in the optimal position above the body of C2 vertebra. Any deviation from this alignment indicates either ligamentous disruption or a broken vertebra.

Ask yourself three important questions:

1. Do the lateral margins of C1 align vertically with the adjacent lateral margins of C2?

2. Are the spaces on each side of the Peg approximately equal?

3. Is there a fracture line across the base of the Peg?

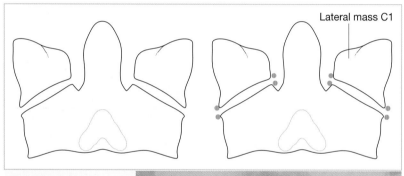

Lateral mass C1

Question 1.

We teach that a more relevant name for the Peg view is:

"The lining up of the lateral masses view".

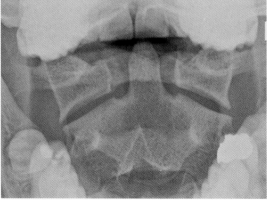

Normal anatomy of the C1–C2 articulation. Looking down from above.

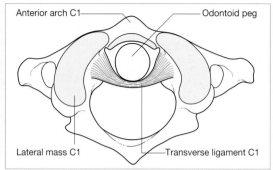

Anterior arch C1 — Odontoid peg

Lateral mass C1 — Transverse ligament C1

If the lateral masses do not align vertically, then there could be several possible explanations.

First consider subluxation due to ligament rupture.

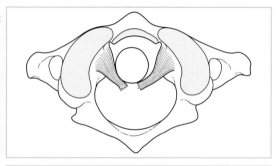

Second, consider fracture of the body of C1; either isolated to a single lateral mass or to a burst fracture of C1 (a Jefferson fracture).

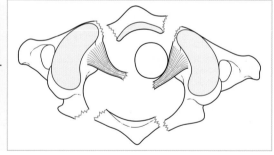

Finally, consider a developmental variation or just simple rotation of a normal neck (see p. 182), as shown on this AP Peg view.

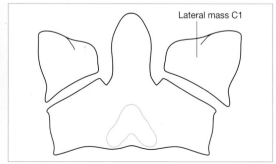

Lateral mass C1

**Question 2:
Frequent pitfall.**

Slight rotation of the neck may cause the space on each side of the Peg to appear unequal. However, if the lateral masses of C1 and C2 remain normally aligned then the asymmetry can be attributed to rotation rather than indicating damage to the transverse ligament (p. 191).

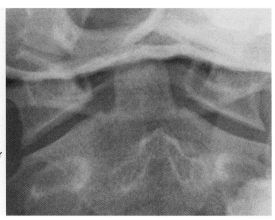

**Question 2:
Pitfall.**

Occasionally, asymmetric alignment of a lateral mass will be present; ie the edges of the adjacent C1/C2 lateral masses do not line up perfectly. This might suggest vertebral subluxation. However, non-pathological causes for this finding do occur: either some slight positional rotation of the neck, or a developmental variation in the size of the C1 and C2 lateral masses[1,12–14]. In most instances it is fairly easy to decide whether an offset on one side of the C1–C2 articulation is simply developmental… just check whether there is any offset on the other side. If the lateral masses line up normally on the other side then developmental asymmetry is the likely explanation.

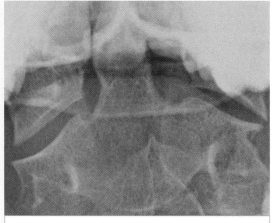

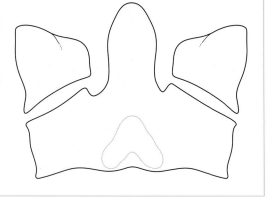

Question 3:
Pitfall — the Mach effect.

It is very common to see a thin black line crossing the base of the Peg or the top of the Peg. This is an optical illusion[15] resulting from the overlapping shadows of superimposed structures. This line is known as a Mach band or a Mach effect. Be aware of this line.

But, be careful...

The inexperienced observer should always seek advice before too readily dismissing any line in this area as a Mach artefact.

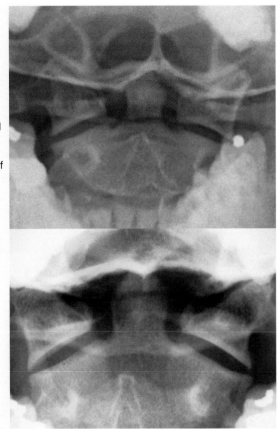

Another artefact.

The apparent vertical fracture through the Peg is an artefact. It is caused by the gap between two of the teeth (incisors).

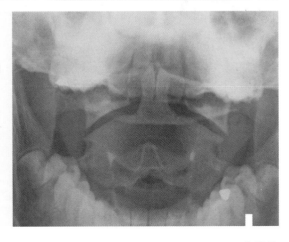

Cervical spine

Priority 3: Long AP view checklist

The lateral and Peg views are the most useful images. The diagnostic return from the long AP view, in terms of abnormalities detected, will be considerably less. In addition, it is easy for the unwary to read too much into the AP view.

Ask yourself two questions:

1. Are the spinous processes in a straight line?
    If not, consider unilateral facet joint dislocation (see p. 194).

2. Is the space between adjacent spinous processes approximately equal?

A warning: if a space is more than 50% wider than the space immediately above or below, this is highly suggestive of an anterior cervical dislocation[16]. In practice this observation is most useful in the severely injured patient whose shoulders have obscured some of the vertebrae on the lateral radiograph[17]. It can provide an important warning that the neck must be managed very carefully until a lateral view or CT has accurately defined the alignment of the vertebrae.

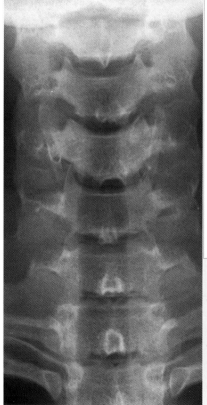

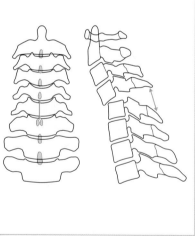

The normal radiograph shows the spinous processes in a straight line.

The C4 and C5 spinous processes are bifid and bifid processes are a very common occurrence.

The drawings illustrate how an anterior dislocation can result in a large gap between the spinous processes at the affected level.

184

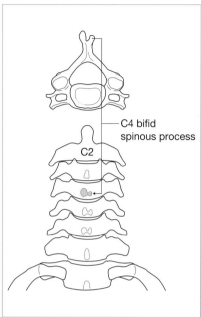

— C4 bifid
spinous process

C2

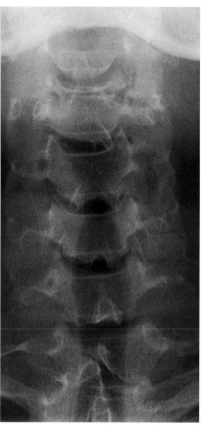

Question 1: Pitfall.

Sometimes a bifid spinous process
(a normal variant) might suggest that
the processes are not in a straight line.

This normal radiograph shows bifid
processes at all levels.

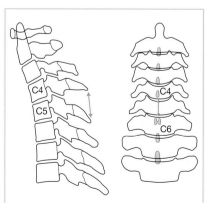

C4
C5

C4
C6

**Question 2:
Pitfall.**

If muscle spasm causes the neck to be
held in flexion then the 50% rule does
not apply.

Whenever the 50% rule (p. 184) is broken
you must check the lateral view again in
order to see whether or not neck flexion
or a dislocation is the explanation for the
increase in space on the AP radiograph.

The common injuries

Injuries at C1

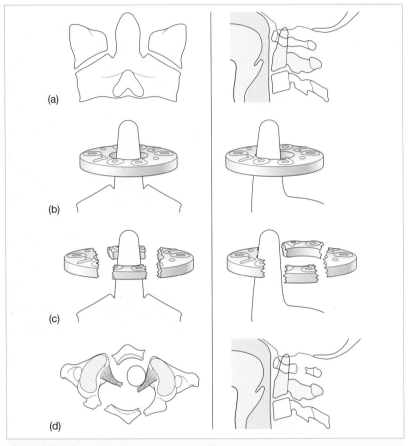

(a)

(b)

(c)

(d)

The C1 (Atlas) vertebra is a vulnerable structure.

(a) Normal appearances of the C1–C2 articulation on the AP Peg view and on the lateral view.

(b) C1 is a thin and insubstantial bone (rather like a Polo mint or a Life Saver).

(c) A vertical (ie axial) force can shatter this Polo mint. Examples include: a heavy weight falling on the top of the head; the skull hitting the bottom of an empty swimming pool.

(d) A vertical force can fracture C1 in several positions (a Jefferson fracture). Sometimes the transverse ligament (situated across the posterior aspect of the odontoid peg) can rupture. On occasion high impact forces (not necessarily vertical) will cause the transverse ligament to rupture on its own.

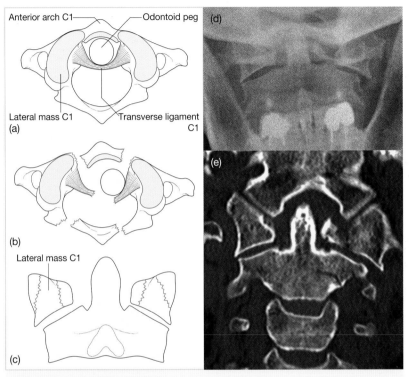

Anterior arch C1 — Odontoid peg (d)

Lateral mass C1 — Transverse ligament C1
(a)

(b)

Lateral mass C1
(c)

(e)

Jefferson fracture: C1 vertebra

(a) A normal C1 vertebra viewed from above.

(b) A vertical (axial) force has shattered the C1 vertebra and caused a rupture of the transverse ligament.

(c) The appearance of (b) as it would be seen on an AP Peg view. The main finding is the displacement of the C1 lateral masses on the right side—ie they do not line up with the lateral masses of the C2 vertebra. The fracture lines might not be easy to identify.

(d) Radiograph of a patient struck on the top of the head by a violent vertical force. There is a unilateral (left-sided) Jefferson fracture. This Peg view shows that the lateral masses of C1 and C2 on the patient's left side do not line up. Also, there is fragmentation of the left lateral mass of the C1 vertebra. The CT scan (e) confirms these findings (and also shows an additional undisplaced fracture of the C2 vertebra).

Cervical spine

Injuries at C2 involving the Peg

Evidence from the lateral view

- A line (fracture) crossing the Peg. Usually seen across its base.

- Any misalignment in the anterior or posterior cortex of C2.

- Any break in the anterior or the posterior margin of Harris' ring (p. 176).

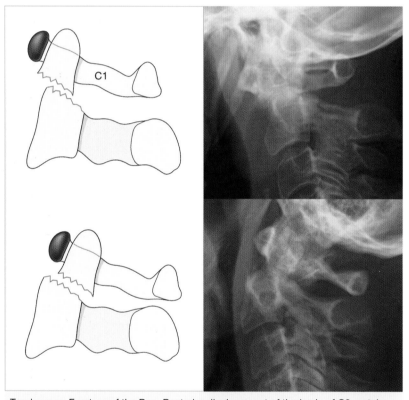

Top images: Fracture of the Peg. Posterior displacement of the body of C2 vertebra.

Bottom image: Fracture of the Peg. Anterior displacement of the body of C2 vertebra.

The key to diagnosis is understanding the normal anatomy.

Confused? Start by identifying the anterior arch of the C1 vertebra (ie the "coffee bean", p. 175). The coffee bean is an easily identifiable landmark that is present on all radiographs. The normal Peg should be positioned immediately behind the coffee bean. The anterior aspect of the normal Peg should continue inferiorly as the anterior cortex of the body of C2 vertebra.

Evidence from the Peg view

- A line crossing the base of the Peg (beware Mach band artefacts, p. 183).

- A Peg that is not vertical (ie it is tilted to the left or to the right).

- In practice the AP Peg view rarely discloses a Peg fracture easily—the lateral radiograph is the crucial view to rely on.

A base of Peg fracture.

Often very difficult to diagnose on the AP Peg view.

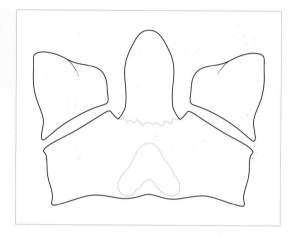

Sometimes a fractured Peg will lean to one side.

Apply this aphorism:

"A leaning Peg is a bad Peg"

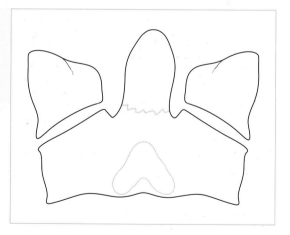

Cervical spine

Injuries involving the body or the posterior elements of C2

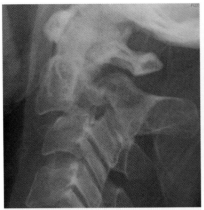

C2 Hangman's fracture[8].

A bilateral fracture through the pars interarticularis of C2 vertebra. Unstable injury caused by hyperextension. Historically consequent on hanging. Now typically results from a motor vehicle accident with (eg) the forehead striking the dashboard. In this patient there is also a fracture of the body of C3.

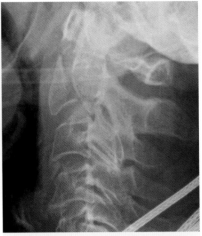

Oblique fracture through the body of the C2 vertebra.

Sometimes this causes the anterior-posterior width of the body of C2 to be increased[18] (the so-called "Fat C2" sign).

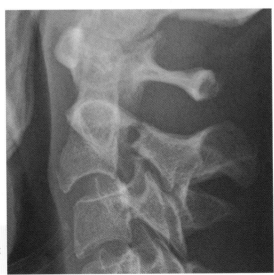

C2 Hangman's fracture with anterior displacement of C2 on C3 vertebra.

C2 subluxation due to rupture of the transverse ligament

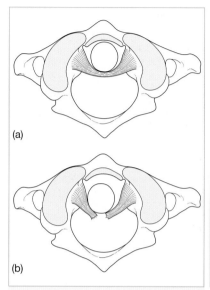

(a)

(b)

The transverse ligament viewed from above. (a) = normal, (b) = ruptured.

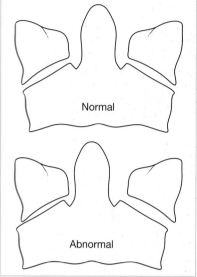

Normal

Abnormal

Ruptured ligament: Evidence from the Peg view. Check the margins of the lateral masses of C1 and C2. If all four lateral masses do not line up in a normal manner then a rupture of the ligament is probable. A Jefferson fracture (p. 186) is an alternative possibility.

Ruptured ligament: Evidence from the lateral view.

The space between the anterior arch of C1 (the "coffee bean") and the anterior aspect of the Peg must not exceed 3 mm in adults.

In this patient the space is approximately 7 mm. C2 has subluxed posteriorly because the transverse ligament has ruptured.

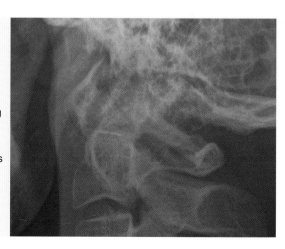

Cervical spine

Fractures C3–C7

Including spinous process fracture, vertebral body compression fracture, and hyperflexion teardrop fracture.

The cardinal rule: The lateral radiograph must always, always, include a well visualised superior surface of the T1 vertebra. Many errors[1,3,5] occur because the top of T1 has not been included on the radiograph. Check the lateral view as described on p. 174.

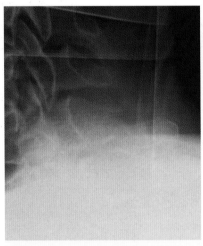

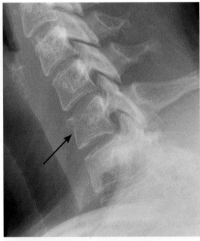

C7 spinous process fracture. This is evidence of major violence. Important ligaments are likely to be torn.

C7 vertebral body compression fracture (arrow). Consequent on a flexion injury.

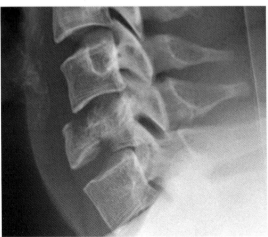

C6 hyperflexion teardrop fracture.

Consequent on extreme flexion and axial loading. An unstable injury.

Subluxations/dislocations C3–C7

Anterior subluxation.

A flexion-rotation injury. Recognition is usually easy. Detected when there is disruption—at any level—of the three arcs described on page 178. Sometimes it is a single arc that appears most out of line.

Subluxed mid-cervical vertebra with arc disruption.

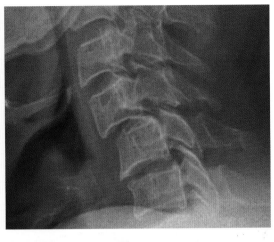

Unilateral facet joint dislocation.

Consequent on a distraction–flexion force with a rotational element. Commonly overlooked on radiographs.

Look for:

- AP view: spinous processes out of line.

- Lateral view: 10–20% forward subluxation (at the C6/C7 level in this patient).

Then:

- Obtain the opinion of an experienced observer.

- Confirmation of this very precise diagnosis requires the judgement of an expert.

Cervical spine

Explaining unilateral facet joint dislocation

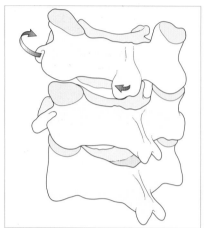

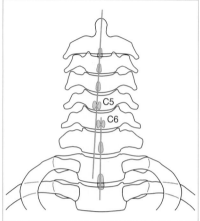

The facet of one vertebra has jumped forwards off the facet of the vertebra below. The jump occurs on one side only.

The rotational displacement at the facet joint causes the spinous processes to be out of line on the AP view.

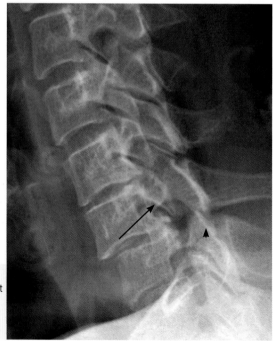

The jumping off of one facet (arrow) from the facet below (arrowhead) results in the forward subluxation on the lateral view.

Pitfalls

On the AP Peg view

- An unequal space on each side of the Peg is commonly due to patient positioning with the neck slightly rotated. All the same, such a finding necessitates very careful inspection of the alignment of the lateral masses (see p. 180).

- A black line across the Peg might be a Mach effect or tooth artefact (p. 183) rather than a fracture. Evaluation of the lateral view is then the important next step.

On the long AP view

- A bifid spinous process may falsely suggest that processes are not in line (pp. 184–185).

- If muscle spasm holds the neck in flexion, the 50% rule for normal spacing does not apply (pp. 184–185).

Developmental variants

A vertebra (arrow) may appear slightly narrow anteriorly with loss of the normal square or rectangular outline. This can mimic a compression fracture.

Sometimes this narrowed appearance is due to old trauma. Occasionally it is due to persistence of the normal but slightly wedged shape that is often present during adolescence[19].

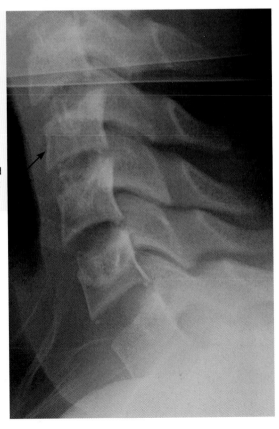

Anterior opacity

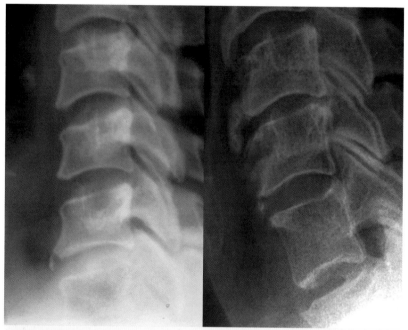

A small calcified opacity anterior to a vertebral body can be mistaken for an avulsed fracture fragment. Sometimes it is simply a remnant of an old secondary ossification centre[19] (left). An age related osteophyte can also produce a similar appearance (right). When such an opacity is detected, an experienced observer should review the radiographs.

Spasm related—delayed instability

Following trauma, severe pain and spasm may make it difficult to exclude a significant injury to the posterior ligament complex. Muscle spasm can hold the neck in an anatomical position and mask ligamentous rupture. Instability may only become evident after a few days when the spasm has reduced.

It is therefore important that any patient with severe pain and spasm who appears fit for discharge and is put in a collar should be asked to attend again in a few days for further evaluation. Lateral views in flexion and extension might form part of that evaluation. These additional radiographs must be taken under close clinical supervision. If they remain at all equivocal, an MRI examination should be obtained in order to exclude a ligamentous injury.

Age related changes

Age related degenerative changes are very common over the age of 40. Distinguishing between changes due to cervical spondylosis and those resulting from an acute injury is not always easy.

The age related appearances shown below are frequently present in the middle-aged and the elderly.

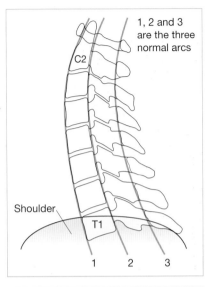

1, 2 and 3 are the three normal arcs

C2

Shoulder

T1

1   2   3

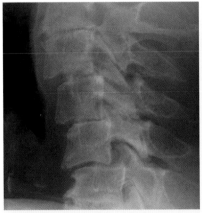

Anterior subluxation of a vertebra secondary to facet joint degenerative change (at several levels on this radiograph). There is no simple way of distinguishing this from traumatic subluxation. In most cases, correlation of the clinical symptoms and signs with the site of the radiographic abnormality will provide reassurance. In some cases an injury should be assumed until an experienced observer has reviewed the radiographs[20].

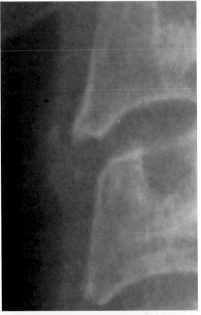

A step in the anterior vertebral line. The step is due to a protruding anterior osteophyte. It might be misinterpreted as indicating vertebral subluxation.

197

References

1. Richards PJ. Cervical spine clearance: a review. Injury 2005; 36: 248–269.
2. Anekstein Y, Jeroukhimov I, Bar-Ziv Y et al. The use of dynamic CT surview for cervical spine clearance in comatose trauma patients: a pilot prospective study. Injury 2008; 39: 339–346.
3. Daffner RH, Sciulli RL, Rodriguez A et al. Imaging for evaluation of suspected cervical spine trauma: a 2 year analysis. Injury 2006; 37: 652–658.
4. Goldberg W, Mueller C, Panacek E et al. Distribution and patterns of blunt traumatic cervical spine injury. Ann Emerg Med 2001; 38: 17–21.
5. Tins BJ, Cassar-Pullicino VN. Imaging of acute cervical spine injuries: review and outlook. Clin Rad 2004; 59: 865–880.
6. Mann FA, Kubal WS, Blackmore CC. Improving the imaging diagnosis of cervical spine injury in the very elderly: implications of the epidemiology of injury. Emerg Radiol 2000; 7: 36–41.
7. Harris JH, Burke JT, Ray RD et al. Low (type III) odontoid fractures: a new radiographic sign. Radiology 1984; 153: 353–356.
8. Harris JH, Mirvis SE. The radiology of acute cervical spine trauma. 3rd ed. Williams & Wilkins, 1996.
9. Harris JH. The cervicocranium: its radiographic assessment. Radiology 2001; 218: 337–351.
10. Herr CH, Ball PA, Sargent SK, Quinton HB. Sensitivity of prevertebral soft tissue measurement at C3 for detection of cervical spine fractures and dislocations. Am J Emerg Med 1998; 16: 346–349.
11. Matar LD, Doyle AJ. Prevertebral soft-tissue measurements in cervical spine injury. Austr Radiol 1997; 41: 229–237.
12. Gehweiler JA Jr, Daffner RH, Roberts L Jr. Malformations of the atlas vertebra simulating the Jefferson fracture. Am J Roentgenol 1983; 140: 1083–1086.
13. Suss RA, Zimmerman RD, Leeds NE. Pseudospread of the atlas: false sign of Jefferson fracture in young children. Am J Roentgenol 1983; 140: 1079–1082.
14. Mirvis SE. How much lateral atlantodental interval asymmetry and atlantoaxial lateral mass asymmetry is acceptable on an open-mouth odontoid radiograph, and when is additional investigation necessary? Am J Roentgenol 1998; 170: 1106–1107.
15. Daffner RH. Pseudofracture of the dens: Mach bands. Am J Roentgenol 1977; 128: 607–612.
16. Naidich JB, Naidich TP, Garfein C et al. The widened interspinous distance: a useful sign of anterior cervical dislocation in the supine frontal projection. Radiology 1977; 123: 113–116.
17. Harris JH, Yeakley JS. Radiographically subtle soft tissue injuries of the cervical spine. Curr Prob Diagn Radiol 1989; 18: 161–190.
18. Pellei DD. The fat C2 sign. Radiology 2000; 217: 359–360.
19. Keats TE, Anderson MW. Atlas of normal Roentgen variants that may simulate disease. 9th ed. Elsevier, 2012.
20. Lee C, Woodring JH, Rogers LF, Kim KS. The radiographic distinction of degenerative slippage (spondylolisthesis and retrolisthesis) from traumatic slippage of the cervical spine. Skeletal Radiol 1986; 15: 439–443.

12

Thoracic & lumbar spine

Normal anatomy

Analysis: the checklists

The common injury

Less frequent but important injuries

Pitfalls

Regularly overlooked injuries

▤ Transverse process fractures.

The standard radiographs

Lateral and **AP** views.

Abbreviations

AP, anterior-posterior; L1, the 1st lumbar vertebra; T6, the 6th thoracic vertebra.

Normal anatomy

Lateral view—thoracic and lumbar vertebrae[1-4]

- The vertical contour of the lumbar spine is a smooth unbroken arc.

- The vertebral bodies are the same height anteriorly and posteriorly.

- The posterior margin of each vertebral body is slightly concave.

- Each vertebra is intact —ie no step, no break, no kinking.

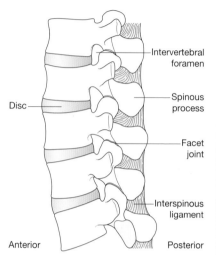

Disc

Intervertebral foramen

Spinous process

Facet joint

Interspinous ligament

Anterior

Posterior

The three column spine

The concept of a three column spine[1] is a familiar one when evaluating a CT or MRI examination. This anatomical concept can also be applied to the lateral radiograph.

- **Anterior column**
  The anterior longitudinal ligament, the anterior part of the annulus fibrosus, and the anterior two thirds of the vertebral body.

- **Middle column**
  The posterior longitudinal ligament, the posterior part of the annulus fibrosus, and the posterior margin of the vertebral body.

- **Posterior column**
  The facet joints, the pedicles, and the posterior ligaments.

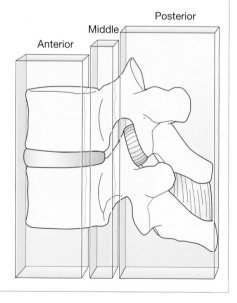

Posterior

Middle

Anterior

AP view—thoracic vertebrae

In the thoracic spine the soft tissue shadow of the left paraspinal line (aka paravertebral stripe) should be closely applied to the vertebral bodies. This line is produced by the interface between the paravertebral soft tissues and the adjacent lung.

On the right side there is no visible paraspinal line[5,6].

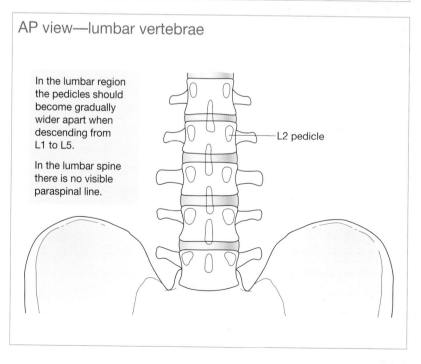

Pedicle

Transverse process

Spinous process

Descending aorta

Paraspinal line

AP view—lumbar vertebrae

In the lumbar region the pedicles should become gradually wider apart when descending from L1 to L5.

In the lumbar spine there is no visible paraspinal line.

L2 pedicle

Analysis: the checklists

- A step-by-step analytical approach when evaluating the plain films may provide an immediate indication that a potentially catastrophic injury has occurred.

- The AP projection can provide useful information, but the lateral radiograph is invariably the more useful. 70–90% of detectable plain film abnormalities will be shown on the lateral projection[7,8]. Also, it is the lateral radiograph to which the three column stability principle[1-3] is applied:

> *"Instability is present if any two of the three columns are disrupted"*

On the lateral view

Look for:

- Loss of height or wedging of a vertebral body: this is evidence of a compression fracture. Wedging may be associated with loss of the normal concavity of the posterior aspect of the vertebral body[9]. This loss indicates significant posterior displacement of the middle column.

- Fragment(s) of bone detached from the anterior aspect of a vertebral body.

- More than one abnormality. The importance of recognising all of the radiological abnormalities that may be present is explained under stability (pp. 209–210).

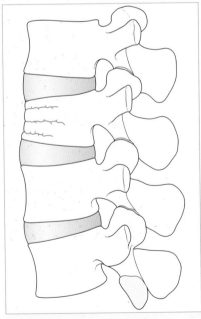

Wedge compression fracture of a lumbar vertebra.

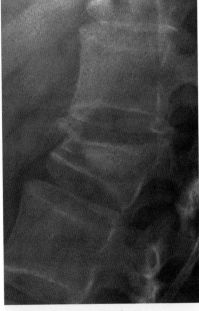

L1 wedge compression fracture.

202

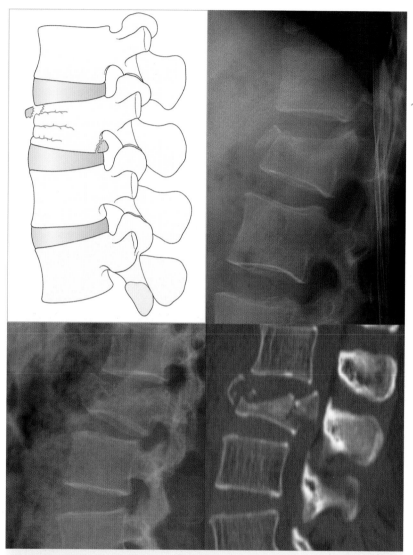

Wedge compression fractures.

- Top left: two fragments have been detached. Two columns are disrupted... the anterior and middle columns. Unstable.

- Top right: Several fragments. The posterior margin of L1 is disrupted and bulges into the spinal canal. Two column disruption. Unstable.

- Bottom left and right: Large fragment in canal. Two columns disrupted. Unstable.

Thoracic & lumbar spine

On the AP view

Thoracic spine

Look for:

■ Localised displacement or widening of the thoracic paraspinal lines. In the context of trauma, displacement or bulging should be regarded as indicating a paraspinal haematoma resulting from a vertebral body fracture.

Thoracic and/or lumbar spine

Look for:

■ Abnormal widening of the distance between the pedicles. This indicates that vertebral fragments have splayed apart.

■ Fracture of a transverse process. This can be subtle; careful windowing on the digital images will usually be necessary.

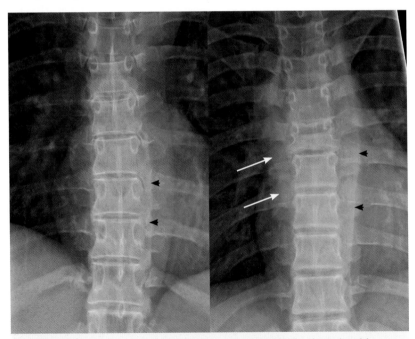

The image on the left is normal. Note that the left paraspinal line (arrowheads) parallels the lateral margin of the vertebral bodies. Further laterally, is the vertical shadow of the descending aorta.

The image on the right is abnormal. There is a bulge of the left paraspinal line (arrowheads) caused by a haematoma resulting from the fracture of T6 vertebra. The haematoma has caused the right paravertebral stripe to appear as a bulge (arrows) in this patient. Normally, the right paravertebral stripe is not visible.

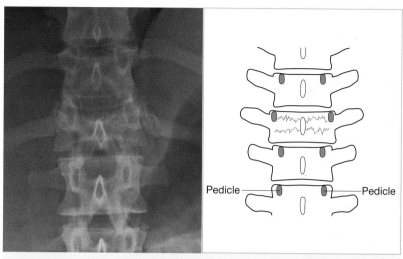

Left: T12 fracture. The vertebra has lost height. Note that the pedicles have been splayed apart. Right: fracture of a lumbar vertebra. The pedicles have been splayed apart. Normally, the pedicles gradually splay apart very slightly from L1 to L5, but there should not be any sudden widening as shown here.

Fractures of the right-sided transverse processes of L2, L3, and L4 vertebrae (arrows).

Most commonly these fractures result from rotation or extreme lateral bending.

Helpful hint: In the context of high energy trauma (and multiple injuries) the detection of transverse process fractures should raise the possibility of a major injury lower in the lumbosacral spine. See "sentinel sign", p. 211.

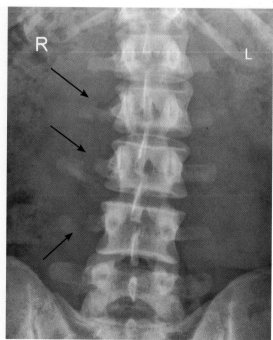

The common injury

There is only one common—ie regularly occurring—vertebral fracture.

Osteoporotic compression fractures[10].

- ☐ Vertebral compression fractures are common in an ageing population.

- ☐ Many/most of these fractures are clinically silent. Approximately 30% of people sustaining a fracture will be symptomatic and usually present with back pain.

- ☐ Radiologically the appearance on the lateral radiograph is that of a wedge compression fracture.

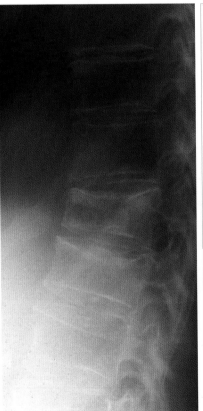

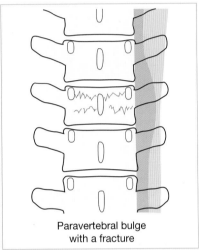

Paravertebral bulge
with a fracture

**Compression fracture
of a mid thoracic vertebra.**

In this example a haematoma bulges the left paravertebral stripe. In practice such a haemorrhagic bulge is rare unless high energy trauma has occurred.

Elderly patient with severe back pain.

Compression fractures (vertebral flattening) of T11 and T12 vertebrae.

Less frequent but important injuries

Fractures following trauma

These important injuries are all consequent on high energy trauma. The forces acting at the time of a particular injury can be very complex.

Assessment:

▤ First, look for distinct fracture patterns.

▤ Second, assess stability by evaluating the three columns.

Distinct fracture patterns...

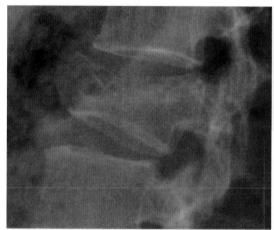

Flexion compression injury (wedge fracture) of L2 vertebra.

Radiological pattern: The anterior aspect of the vertebral body loses height, but the posterior part does not.

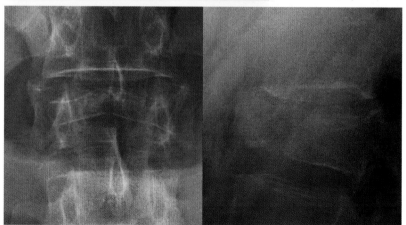

Vertical compression injury (burst fracture) of L1 vertebra.

Radiological pattern: Severe comminution and flattening of a vertebral body. Often caused by a fall from a height and landing on the feet.

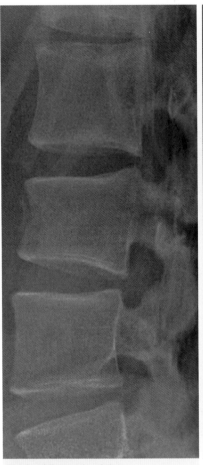

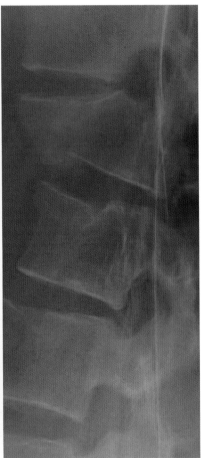

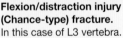

Flexion/distraction injury (Chance-type) fracture.
In this case of L3 vertebra.

Radiological pattern: This is a shearing injury. Various patterns occur[11,12].

One fairly common pattern:
The vertebral body fractures transversely, with the spinous process and the postero-superior aspect of the vertebral body also fractured. Classically a head-on car crash with the upper torso hurled forwards whilst the pelvis is held by a lap seat belt.

Fracture dislocation injury. In this case affecting the T12/L1 level. (Additional vertebral fractures are also evident.)

Radiological pattern:
A fracture and subluxation (or dislocation) of one vertebra on another.

Assessing stability by evaluating the three columns...

When a radiographic abnormality is detected it needs to be categorised as showing either a stable or an unstable appearance. Assess each of the three columns on the lateral radiograph (p. 200). In general, the term 'stable injury' should only be applied to minimal/moderate compression fractures with an intact posterior column.

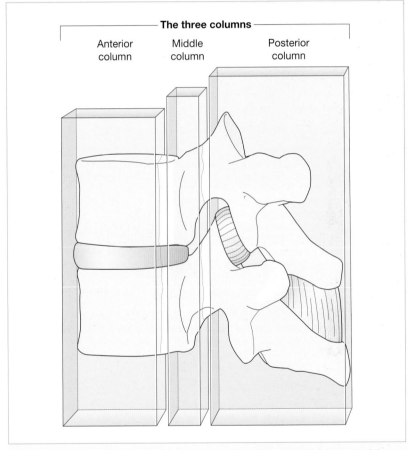

The three columns are normal in this illustration. The alignment, the shape, and the contours of these vertebrae are seen to be anatomical. The assessment of each column on every lateral radiograph is a most important task. If a disruption of any two of the three columns is detected then the injury will be classified as unstable.

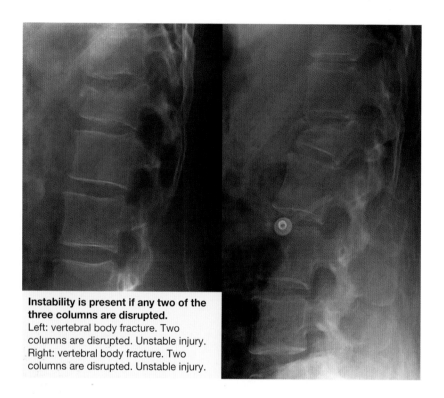

Instability is present if any two of the three columns are disrupted.
Left: vertebral body fracture. Two columns are disrupted. Unstable injury.
Right: vertebral body fracture. Two columns are disrupted. Unstable injury.

Stability following high energy trauma

Wedge fracture.	Many are stable. Nevertheless, the clinical significance of a particular wedge fracture may be underestimated. These fractures will occasionally cause middle column bone fragments to intrude into the spinal canal.
Burst fracture	Invariably unstable.
Chance-type fracture:	Unstable. Usually disrupted posterior and middle columns; frequently, the anterior column is also involved.
Fracture dislocation injury	Highly unstable.
Transverse process fracture	As an isolated finding this is a stable injury.

Pitfalls

The right paraspinal line

This line is situated adjacent to the thoracic vertebrae and it is not seen in normal individuals. There is one exception: it may be visualised in some middle-aged and elderly patients because the pleura is displaced by age-related lateral osteophytes[13]. In these patients the visible right paraspinal line does not signify pathological tissue.

Dismissing transverse process fractures as trivial

If transverse process fractures are seen after high energy trauma. then it is important to assess the lumbosacral junction appearances most carefully[14]. Following severe high energy trauma transverse process fractures may be overlooked, or dismissed as minor, particularly in the presence of pulmonary, abdominal, vascular, or brain injury. Lumbosacral junction dislocation (a rare injury) frequently has fractures of several transverse processes on the AP view. This has given rise to the term "sentinal sign".

Schmorl's nodes[14]

These are focal indentations of the vertebral body end plates seen at all ages but most commonly in younger people. The aetiology of Schmorl's nodes is controversial and their clinical importance remains undecided. They are a relatively common finding in the thoracic and lumbar spine. A Schmorl's node should not be read as an important pathological finding.

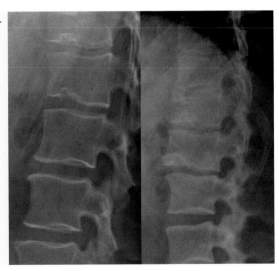

Two patients with irregular indentations on the end plates of several vertebral bodies. Schmorl's nodes.

References

1. Denis F. The three column spine and its significance in the classification of acute thoracolumbar spinal injuries. Spine 1983; 8: 817–831.
2. Murphey MD, Batnitzky S, Bramble JM. Diagnostic imaging of spinal trauma. Radiol Clin North Am 1989; 27: 855–872.
3. Pathria MN, Petersilge CA. Spinal trauma. Radiol Clin North Am 1991; 29: 847–865.
4. Vialle R, Charosky S, Rillardon L et al. Traumatic dislocation of the lumbosacral junction diagnosis, anatomical classification and surgical strategy. Injury 2007; 38: 169–181.
5. Genereux GP. The posterior pleural reflections. Am J Roentgenol 1983; 141: 141–149.
6. Donnelly LF, Frush DP, Zheng J et al. Differentiating normal from abnormal inferior thoracic paravertebral soft tissues on chest radiography in children. Am J Roentgenol 2000; 175: 477–483.
7. Berquist TH. Imaging of orthopedic trauma. 2nd ed. Lippincott Williams & Wilkins, 1992.
8. Gehweiler JA, Osborne RL, Becker RF. The radiology of vertebral trauma. WB Saunders, 1980.
9. Daffner RH, Deeb ZL, Rothfus WE. The posterior vertebral body line: importance in the detection of burst fractures. Am J Roentgenol 1987; 148: 93–96.
10. Prather H, Watson JO, Gilula LA. Nonoperative management of osteoporotic vertebral compression fractures. Injury 2007; 38 (3): S40–S48.
11. Bernstein MP, Mirvis SE, Shanmuganathan K. Chance-type fractures of the thoracolumbar spine: imaging analysis in 53 patients. Am J Roentgenol 2006; 187: 859–868.
12. Groves CJ, Cassar-Pullicino VN, Tins BJ et al. Chance-type flexion-distraction injuries in the thoracolumbar spine: MR imaging characteristics. Radiology 2005; 236: 601–608.
13. de Lacey G, Morley S, Berman L. The Chest X-Ray: A Survival Guide. Elsevier, 2008.
14. Pfirrmann CW, Resnick D. Schmorl nodes of the thoracic and lumbar spine: radiographic-pathologic study of prevalence, characterization, and correlation with degenerative changes of 1,650 spinal levels in 100 cadavers. Radiology 2001; 219: 368–374.

13

Pelvis

Normal anatomy

Analysis: the checklist

Common fractures, high-energy

Common fractures, low-energy

Sports injuries

Pitfalls

Regularly overlooked injuries

- Undisplaced acetabular fracture.
- Detached acetabular fragment in a patient with a dislocated hip.
- Sacral fractures.
- Avulsed apophysis from the proximal femur or from the innominate bone.

The standard radiograph

AP view.

Abbreviations

AIIS, anterior inferior iliac spine; AP, anterior-posterior; ASIS, anterior superior iliac spine; RTA, road traffic accident; SI joint, sacro-iliac joint.

Normal anatomy

Normal AP view

The pelvis comprises three bone rings:

▓ The main pelvic ring

▓ Two smaller rings formed by the pubic and ischial bones

The robust sacro-iliac joints and the pubic symphysis are part of the main bone ring. The sacro-iliac joints are the strongest joints in the body and resist the normal vertical and anterior-posterior displacement forces; the pubic symphysis is the weakest link in the pelvic ring[1-4].

Arcuate lines are visible as smooth curved borders on the radiograph. They outline the roofs of the sacral formina.

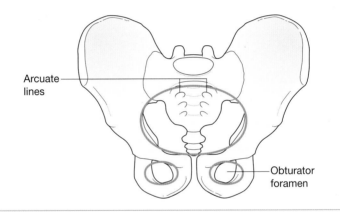

Arcuate lines

Obturator foramen

Developing skeleton: Synchondroses

In children the synchondrosis (cartilaginous junction) between each ischial and pubic bone can sometimes appear confusing. In early childhood these unfused junctions may simulate fracture lines. Subsequently, between the ages of five and seven years, they may mimic healing fractures.

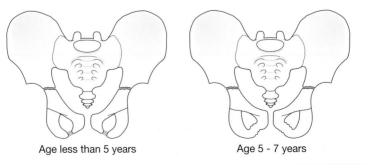

Age less than 5 years

Age 5 - 7 years

Developing skeleton: Pelvic bone apophyses[5–7]

In adolescents and young adults the pelvis shows several small secondary centres (the apophyses). These should be radiographically identical on the two sides.

Apophyses are secondary centres that contribute to the eventual shape, size, and contour of the bone but not to its length. These centres are traction epiphyses as muscles originate from or insert into them. They are vulnerable to severe and acute muscle contraction, and also to repetitive forceful muscle pulls when jumping, hurdling, turning suddenly, or—occasionally—when dancing.

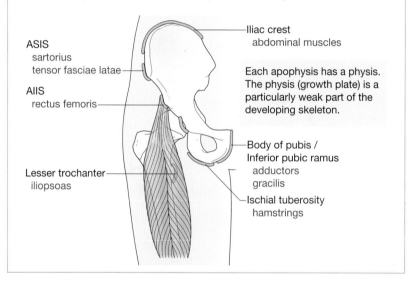

ASIS
sartorius
tensor fasciae latae

AIIS
rectus femoris

Lesser trochanter
iliopsoas

Iliac crest
abdominal muscles

Each apophysis has a physis. The physis (growth plate) is a particularly weak part of the developing skeleton.

Body of pubis /
Inferior pubic ramus
adductors
gracilis

Ischial tuberosity
hamstrings

Age of appearance and fusion of apophyses at the hip and pelvis (years)[5,7]

Apophysis	First seen on radiograph	Fuses to skeleton
Innominate bone		
AIIS	13–15	16–18
ASIS	13–15	21–25
Ischial tuberosity	13–15	20–25
Iliac crest	13–15	21–25
Femur		
Lesser trochanter	11–12	16–17
Greater trochanter	2–3	16–17

Note that some apophyses remain unfused and normal, but are still vulnerable into the early 20s, well after the growth of the long bones has been completed.

Analysis: the checklist

The AP radiograph

Assess:

1. The main pelvic ring. Scrutinise both the inner and outer contours.

2. The two small rings forming the obturator foramina.

3. The sacro-iliac joints. The widths should be equal.

4. The symphysis pubis. The superior surfaces of the body of each pubic bone should align. The maximum width of the joint should be no more than 5 mm.

5. The sacral foramina. Disruption of any of the smooth arcuate lines indicates a sacral fracture. Compare these arcs on the injured and uninjured sides.

6. The region of the acetabulum. This is a complex area and fractures at this site are easy to overlook[3,8–10]. Compare the injured with the uninjured side.

In adolescents and young adults presenting with hip pain but no history of a violent blow also assess:

7. The apophyses (p. 215).

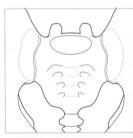

Normal sacro-iliac joints.

Widths approximately equal. The inferior margin of the iliac bone lines up with the inferior aspect of the sacral part of the joint—on both sides.

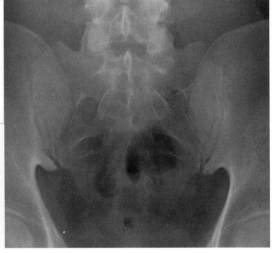

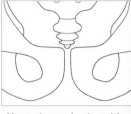

Normal symphysis pubis.

No widening; superior margins at about the same level.

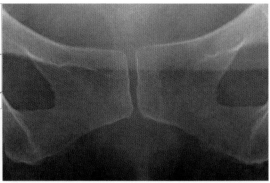

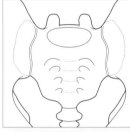

Normal sacral foramina.

The roof of each sacral foramen has a smooth arching superior margin (arrows). No break, no ridge, no irregularity.

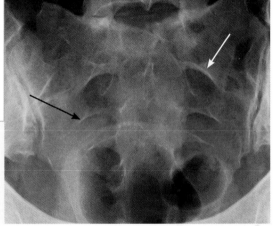

Assessing the apophyses.

Normal. The important finding is that both sides of the pelvis, and both femora, are virtually identical in appearance. There is no significant difference at any site… particularly in the region of each ASIS and AIIS (p. 215).

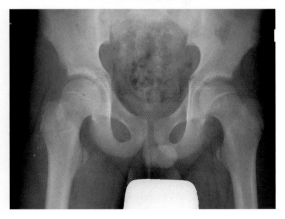

Common fractures, high energy

Fractures involving the main bone ring

A double break in the main pelvic ring is an unstable injury.

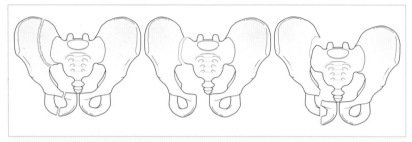

Left: Fracture iliac bone and both pubic rami. Unstable pelvis.

Centre: Bones intact. Ruptured sacro-iliac (SI) joint and diastasis of the pubic symphysis. Unstable pelvis.

Right: Ruptured SI joint and fractures of the pubic rami. Unstable pelvis.

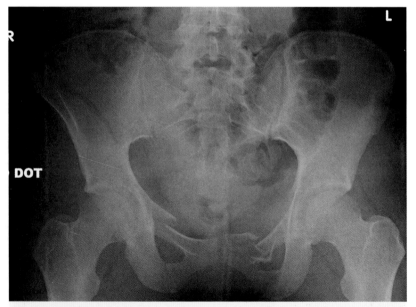

RTA. Note the following fractures: oblique across the right iliac bone; right superior and inferior pubic rami; left superior and inferior pubic rami; body of the left pubic bone. Also, the left SI joint is suspiciously wide. Highly unstable injury.

218

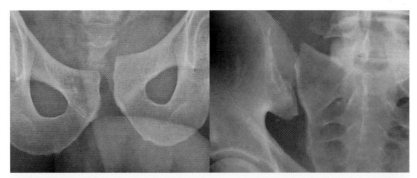

A fracture at one site in a ring is likely to be associated with a disruption of the ring at a second site. The second break might be another fracture or it might be ligamentous disruption at the symphysis pubis (left) or at a SI joint (right).

Acetabular fractures[9,10]

- Frequently sustained by the driver or front seat passenger in a road traffic accident. The patient may complain of pain in the knee as well as in the pelvis.

- A posterior wall fracture is the most frequent acetabular injury.

- Look through the femoral head for evidence of a subtle fracture of the acetabulum. Careful scrutiny is essential. The fracture is frequently comminuted and bone fragments may be trapped within the joint.

- Bone fragments are clinically important. If undetected the consequences may be either difficulty in reduction or premature degenerative change.

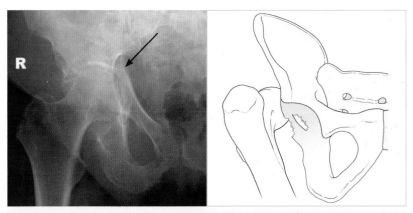

An acetabular fracture (arrow) may result from direct trauma (left) or be associated with a posterior dislocation of the hip (right).

Sacral fractures[1,11]

Often very difficult to detect. The arcuate lines of the sacral foramina need to be carefully assessed, comparing one side with the other.

These fractures are overlooked in as many as 70% of cases. Many sacral fractures are undisplaced, and overlying bowel gas can also obscure these fractures. Additionally, other injuries are often present and these can distract the unwary so that the sacrum is initially overlooked.

A lateral compression force can cause a vertical compression fracture of the sacrum together with accompanying oblique fractures of the pubic rami.

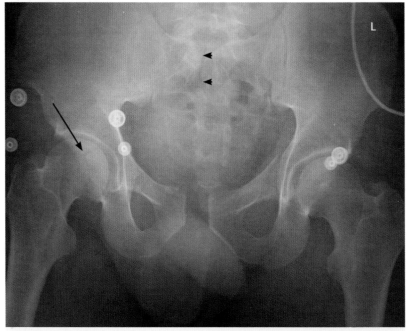

RTA. High energy trauma. Note: diastasis (widening) of the pubic symphysis, fracture of the left superior pubic ramus and an undisplaced fracture through the right acetabulum (arrow). Unless looked for carefully, it is easy to overlook the central fracture through the sacrum (arrowheads); it extends inferiorly from the first sacral segment.

Reminder:
the normal sacrum.

The roof of each foramen (arrows) is smooth— no step, no irregularity.

These smooth curved roofs are often termed the "arcuate lines".

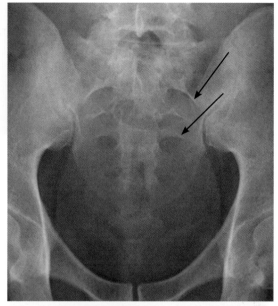

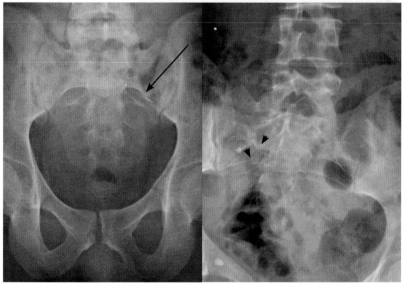

Sacral fractures. Left: Fracture involving the roof of the most superior sacral foramen (arrow) on the left side. Also, a subtle, undisplaced, fracture of the left acetabulum. Right: The roofs of several foramina on the right side are stepped and irregular (arrowheads).

221

Common fractures, low energy

Simple fall in the elderly

Fracture of a pubic ramus or pubic rami. A single fracture of the superior pubic ramus is the commonest pelvic fracture following a fall.

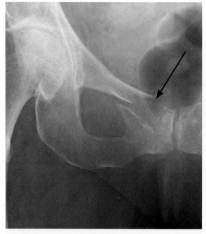

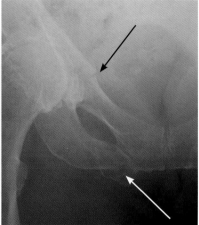

Solitary fracture of the superior pubic ramus (arrow).

Fractures of the superior and inferior pubic rami (arrows).

Injury to the coccyx

History: Fell on buttocks and the coccyx is tender. In practice the radiograph of a normal coccyx may appear angulated and very abnormal. In any case, the radiographic findings do not affect management. Radiography is unnecessary.

Apophyseal avulsion in the young[5,7,12]

These fractures are most commonly caused by repeated or sudden muscle contraction. Avulsions occur during or just after adolescence and not during childhood. Some avulsions can occur during the early 20s when fusion to the main skeleton has yet to occur (see p. 215). Very occasionally a direct blow to an apophysis rather than muscle contraction is the cause of the injury.

Recognition of an apophyseal injury on the plain radiograph will help to avoid additional unnecessary tests and/or inappropriate treatment. Treatment of these injuries is invariably conservative: rest and pain relief.

The most common sites[5,7] of apophyseal avulsion are the ischial tuberosity, the ASIS, the AIIS, and the iliac crest.

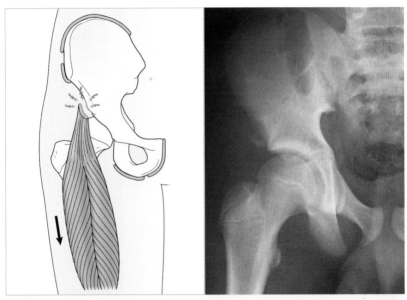

Avulsion of the AIIS apophysis.

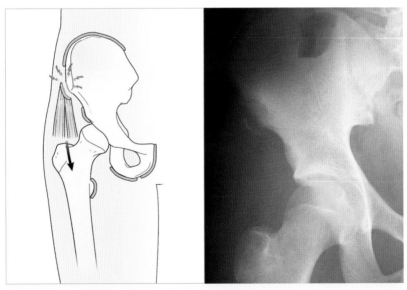

Avulsion of the ASIS apophysis.

Sports injuries: specific avulsions[5–7]

The pelvic apophyses are particularly vulnerable during numerous activities: eg soccer, American football, gymnastics, dance, jumping… ie during any activity that involves rapid acceleration or deceleration, or a sudden change of direction.

An adductor muscle avulsive injury to the apophysis at the pubic symphysis is fairly common in athletes. Radiologically the pubis on the affected side is irregular, and this can extend to involve the inferior pubic ramus.

Avulsion of the lesser trochanter apophysis can occur during vigorous sports, and also when kicking.

"Hip Pointers" are contusions to the iliac crest. Contusions alone do not show major radiographic changes. Avulsion of the lateral part of this apophysis —or entire displacement—has been reported[6].

Sometimes, in an athletic individual, the radiograph will show that more than one apophysis is injured.

History: young athlete with pain in the region of the ischium or the symphysis.

Suspect an apophyseal injury.

- Ischium: insertion of the hamstrings (left).

- Symphysis: insertion of the hip adductors (right).

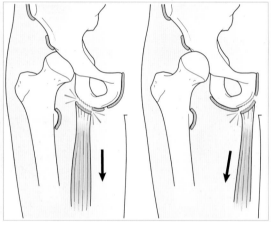

Caution:

- Healing of an avulsion injury may produce considerable ossification/calcification and local deformity. This could be because of wide displacement of the avulsed apophysis or because exuberant calcification is laid down. Do not confuse the appearance with that of a tumour.

- Also, rarefaction of bone or a moth-eaten appearance/lucency at an injured apophysis may be misinterpreted as bone infection or a bone tumour[7,13].

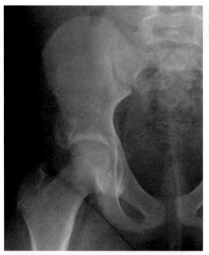

Healing AIIS avulsion.
Profuse callus is present.

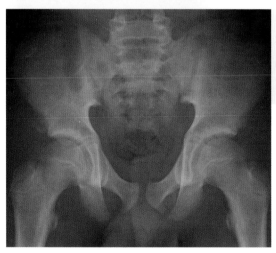

Avulsion of the right AIIS.

The site of the left AIIS appears very slightly rarefied, suspicious of an injury to this apophysis also.

Pitfalls

In adults: Sacral fracture or sacro-illiac joint disruption may be hidden because of patient rotation or by overlying bowel gas.

In children: A normal os acetabuli or an impingement effect (see p. 226) may be misinterpreted as an acute fracture fragment.

Pelvis

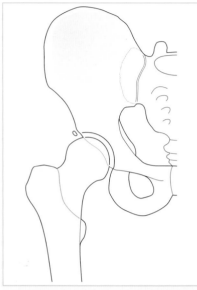 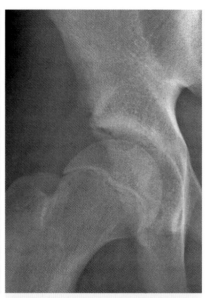

This small fragment of bone is a common finding in children and also in some adults. It is an unfused ossification centre … an os acetabuli. See also p. 242.

The appearance of the lateral aspect of the acetabulum is either an unfused ossification centre (an os acetabuli variant) or an impingement effect[14]. It does not represent an acute fracture.

References

1. Solomon L, Warwick DJ, Nayagam S. Apley's system of orthopaedics and fractures. CRC Press, 2010.
2. Dyer GS, Vrahas MS. Review of the pathophysiology and acute management of haemorrhage in pelvic fracture. Injury 2006; 37: 602–613.
3. MacLeod M, Powell JN. Evaluation of pelvic fractures: clinical and radiologic. Orthop Clin North Am 1997; 28: 299–319.
4. White CE, Hsu JR, Holcomb JB. Haemodynamically unstable pelvic fractures. Injury 2009; 40: 1023–1030.
5. Anderson S. Lower extremity injuries in youth sports. Pediatr Clin North Am 2002; 49: 627–641.
6. Rossi F, Dragoni S. Acute avulsion fractures of the pelvis in adolescent competitive athletes: prevalence, location and sports distribution of 203 cases collected. Skeletal Radiol 2001; 30: 127–131.
7. El-Khoury GY, Daniel WW, Kathol MH. Acute and chronic avulsive injuries. Radiol Clin North Am 1997; 35: 747–766.
8. Theumann NH, Verdon JP, Mouhsine E. Traumatic injuries: imaging of pelvic fractures. Eur Radiol 2002; 12: 1312–1330.
9. Young JW, Burgess AR, Brumback RJ, Poka A. Pelvic fractures: value of plain radiography in early assessment and management. Radiology 1986; 160: 445–451.
10. Durkee NJ, Jacobson J, Jamadar D et al. Classification of common acetabular fractures: radiographic and CT appearances. Am J Roentgenol 2006; 187: 915–925.
11. Robles LA. Transverse sacral fractures: a review. Spine J 2009; 9: 60–69.
12. Sundar M, Carty H. Avulsion fractures of the pelvis in children: a report of 32 fractures and their outcome. Skeletal Radiol 1994; 23: 85–90.
13. Brandser EA, El-Khoury GY, Kathol MH. Adolescent hamstring avulsions that simulate tumors. Emerg Radiol 1995; 2: 273–278.
14. Martinez AE, Li SM, Ganz R, Beck M. Os acetabuli in femoro-acetabular impingement: stress fracture or unfused secondary ossification centre of the acetabular rim? Hip Int 2006; 16: 281–286.

14

Hip
& proximal femur

Normal anatomy

Analysis: the checklists

The common injuries

Uncommon but important injuries

Pitfall

Regularly overlooked injuries

- ▣ Femoral neck fracture
  —minimally displaced.

- ▣ Femoral neck fracture
  —inadequate assessment of the
  lateral radiograph.

- ▣ Pubic ramus fracture.

- ▣ Apophyseal injuries in the young.

The standard radiographs

AP of whole pelvis.
Lateral projection of the painful hip.

Abbreviations

AIIS, anterior inferior iliac spine;
ASIS, anterior superior iliac spine;
CT, computed tomography;
MRI, magnetic resonance imaging;
RTA, road traffic accident;
THR, total hip replacement.

Normal anatomy

AP view

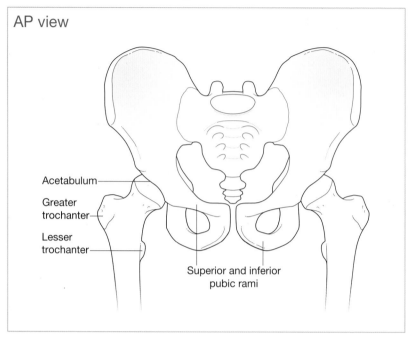

Acetabulum

Greater trochanter

Lesser trochanter

Superior and inferior pubic rami

Lateral view

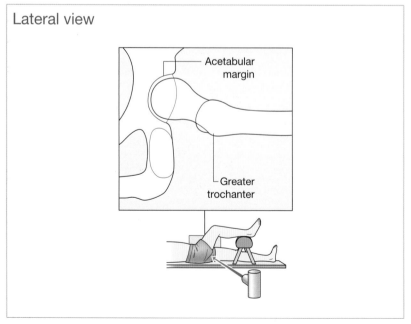

Acetabular margin

Greater trochanter

AP and lateral views

The femoral neck should:

- Have a smooth and intact cortex—no buckle, no step, no ridge.

- Not show any transverse areas of sclerosis.

The intertrochanteric region should:

- Have an appearance identical to the same area on the opposite femur.

- Not show any black or lucent line crossing the intertrochanteric bone nor any interruption in the cortical margin of the greater trochanter.

Secondary centres (apophyses)

The femur and pelvis of an adolescent will show several small secondary centres (the apophyses).

- These should be radiographically identical on the two sides.

- An apophysis contributes to the eventual shape and contour of the bone but not to its overall length. Muscles originate from/insert into the apophyses.

- Each apophysis has a physis. The physis (ie the growth plate) is a particularly weak part of the developing skeleton.

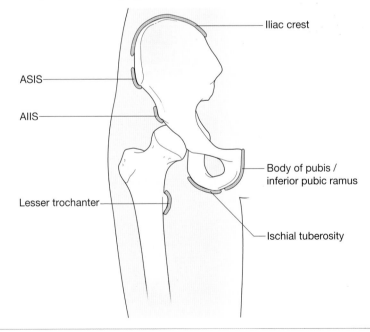

Analysis: the checklists

Detailed inspection should focus on the specific clinical history. Thus…

An elderly patient has suffered a simple fall

Check for:

- A black line—a displaced fracture—across the femoral neck.
- A white line—impacted fracture—in the subcapital region.
- A fracture line through the subcapital region, through the trochanteric region, or through the subtrochanteric region.
- A fracture of a pubic ramus.

A few fractures are very difficult to detect. If the radiographs appear superficially normal it is important to check again and answer the following questions:

- Are the cortical margins of the femoral neck smooth and continuous, or is there a slight step?
- Have I checked the lateral radiograph carefully?

An adolescent patient has acute/chronic pain following athletic activity

Check that:

- The femoral apophyses are similar on the painful and unaffected sides.
- Check the iliac apophyses.

Patient of any age who has sustained high velocity trauma

Check all of the features described above and also check:

- The acetabulum: is it fractured?
- The femoral head: is it dislocated?
- For multiple fractures of the femur and/or the pelvis.

Hip pain in a young patient with no history of recent trauma

- Age 4–10 years: consider Perthe's disease of the femoral head.
- Around the age of puberty: consider slipped capital femoral epiphysis.
- Age 13–25 years: assess all of the femoral and iliac apophyses.
  Chronic repetitive stress can affect the tendinous or muscle attachment at an apophysis and produce soft tissue calcification or an apophyseal irregularity.

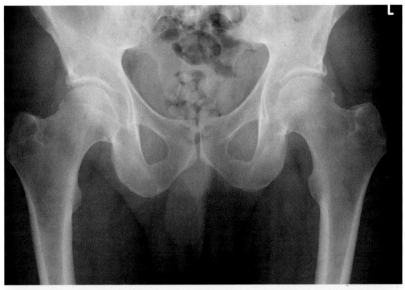

Normal AP view. Injured right hip. The radiographer centres the X-ray beam fairly low so that the proximal shaft of the femur is included. The injured and uninjured sides can be compared.

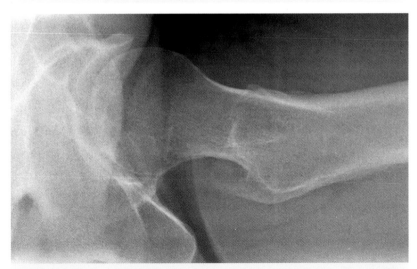

Normal lateral view. The same patient as above. The two sites that must be checked are the neck of the femur and the trochanteric region. This peculiar projection might seem anatomically counterintuitive—see explanation on p. 228.

The common injuries

Elderly patient after a simple fall

Femoral neck fracture

The most common cause of an acute orthopaedic admission in the elderly.
A fall is not always a prerequisite. As the hip twists (eg during a stumble)
a rotational force can occur, causing a fracture through osteoporotic bone.

Fractures of the femoral neck and proximal femur[1,2] occur at characteristic sites.
Approximately 50% of all hip fractures are trochanteric[3].

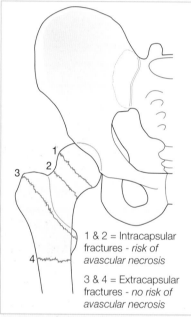

1 & 2 = Intracapsular
fractures - *risk of
avascular necrosis*

3 & 4 = Extracapsular
fractures - *no risk of
avascular necrosis*

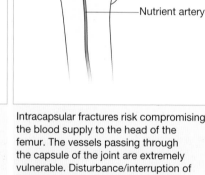

Ligamentum teres
and artery

Capsule

Capsular
artery

Capsular
artery

Nutrient artery

The radiographic findings enable
a fracture of the femoral neck to
be classified as intracapsular or
extracapsular. This classification
has a major impact on determining
the choice of surgical treatment.

Intracapsular fractures risk compromising
the blood supply to the head of the
femur. The vessels passing through
the capsule of the joint are extremely
vulnerable. Disturbance/interruption of
the capsular arteries increases the risk
of non-union or avascular necrosis of
the femoral head. The blood supply is
not similarly affected with an
extracapsular fracture.

Approximately 95% of hip fractures are widely displaced and easy to detect. A few are very difficult to detect. If the radiographs appear superficially normal it is important to check again and answer the following questions:

- Are the cortical margins of the femoral neck really smooth and continuous?

- Is there a black (ie lucent) line crossing the femoral neck?

- Does a dense white line (impaction in a compression fracture) cross the neck?

- Is there any angulation of the neck... compared with the uninjured side?

- Have I checked the lateral radiograph carefully?

Approximately 1% of femoral neck fractures will be undetectable on the initial radiographs[1]. If the radiographs appear normal and there is strong clinical suspicion of a fracture (eg pain on weight bearing) then referral for a same day MRI, CT, or radionuclide examination is indicated. MRI is the preferred investigation.

The fracture that is most frequently missed/overlooked is an undisplaced intracapsular fracture[2].

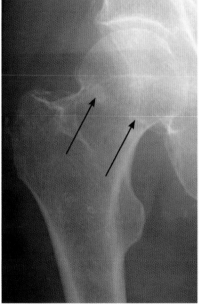

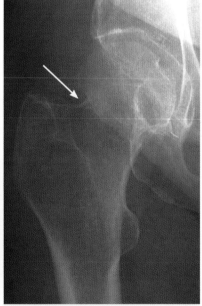

Subcapital fracture.

The white line (arrows) indicates impaction.

Subcapital fracture.

Abnormal angulation (arrow) of the femoral neck is evident.

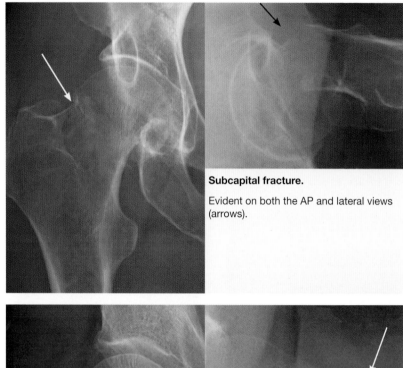

Subcapital fracture.

Evident on both the AP and lateral views (arrows).

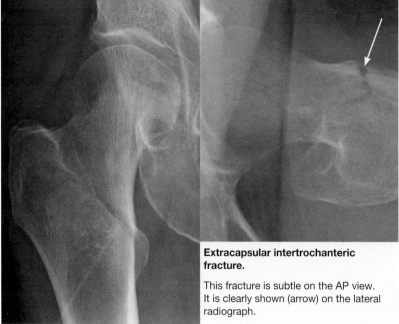

Extracapsular intertrochanteric fracture.

This fracture is subtle on the AP view. It is clearly shown (arrow) on the lateral radiograph.

Pubic ramus fracture

A fracture of a pubic ramus can mimic the symptoms and signs of an undisplaced femoral neck fracture.

Helpful hint: following a simple fall it is rare for a patient to sustain both a femoral neck fracture and a pubic ramus fracture.

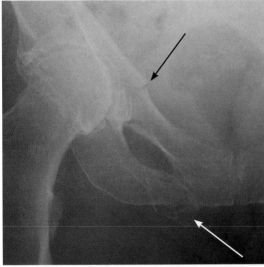

The pubic rami form a ring. Bone rings frequently sustain fractures at two positions (arrows) within the ring.

Always look for two fractures involving the rami.

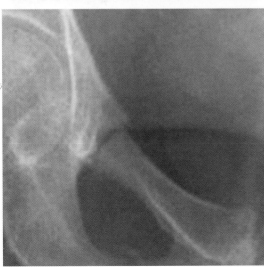

Sometimes there is only one fracture involving the pubic ring. Indeed, the commonest pelvic fracture following a fall in an elderly patient is an isolated fracture of the superior pubic ramus.

235

Adolescent patient with acute hip pain[4,5]

Apophyseal injuries (See also pp. 222–225)

Many of the conditions presenting as acute hip pain in this age group are actually injuries to the pelvis. Always consider an apophyseal injury in a young patient.

Avulsions occur most commonly in sports where a quick burst movement or explosive action occurs. Until the growth centre fuses to the underlying bone (at any time between the ages of 16 and 25 years) an apophysis represents a site of weakness and is vulnerable to forceful muscle contraction. The sites most commonly affected are:

- anterior inferior iliac spine (AIIS)
- anterior superior iliac spine (ASIS)
- ischial tuberosity
- iliac crest.

Always evaluate the iliac apophyses as well as the upper femoral apophyses.

Sometimes bone overgrowth/fragmentation/calcification at the injured site might be initially misinterpreted as indicating a tumour[6].

Clinical impact guideline: treatment of an apophyseal injury is invariably conservative and based on rest and pain relief. Nevertheless, correct diagnosis is still important.

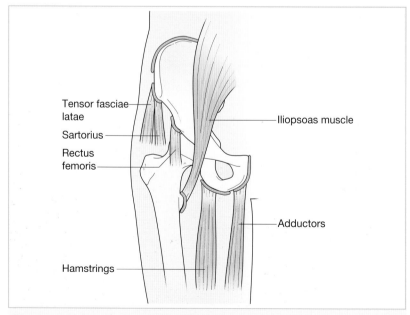

The apophyses and their attached muscles.

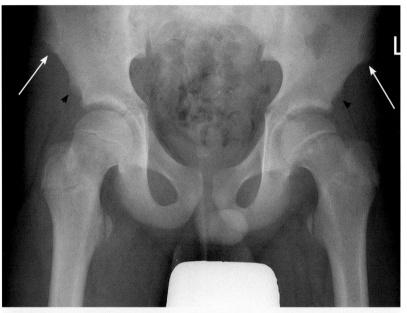

Normal pelvis and hips. Note the normal apophyses in relation to each lesser trochanter. Note the normal appearances at the ASIS (arrows) and the AIIS (arrowheads) on both sides.

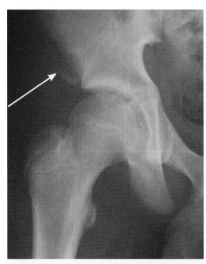

Pain in the hip. The AIIS (arrow) has been avulsed.

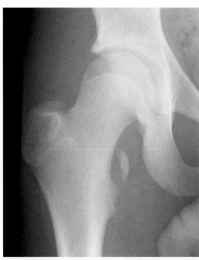

Pain in the hip. Avulsion of an apophysis (lesser trochanter).

Uncommon but important injuries

Acetabular fracture

- A fracture of the acetabulum may produce very similar clinical features to those resulting from an undisplaced fracture of the femoral neck.

- The majority of acetabular fractures result from high energy trauma. Occasionally, a fracture will occur after a simple fall in an individual with severe osteoporosis.

- These fractures are very easy to overlook. Careful scrutiny is essential.

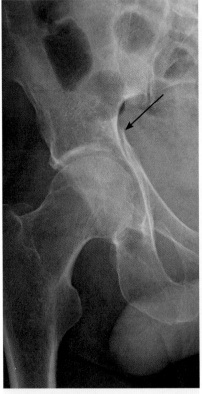

High energy trauma.

Acetabular fracture (arrow).

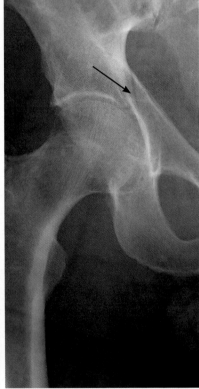

High energy trauma.

Acetabular fracture (arrow).

Dislocations[7,8]

These injuries result from high energy trauma.

Dislocations can be posterior, anterior, or central. Approximately 80% are posterior.

Posterior dislocation.

The extreme force is transmitted up the shaft of the femur, typically in a driver or front seat passenger involved in a road traffic accident (RTA).

The AP view usually demonstrates the dislocation very clearly. The lateral radiograph will confirm the diagnosis.

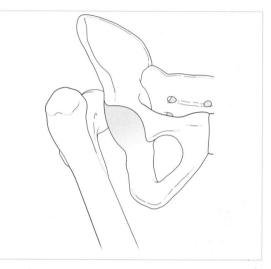

Young male (RTA).

The femoral head is dislocated posteriorly.

A large fragment has been detached from the acetabular margin and lies above the head of the femur. Several other fractures also resulted from the violent impact on this driver at the time of the collision.

Fractures of the acetabular margin are common complications of posterior dislocation.

The incidence of an accompanying acetabular fracture can be as high as 70%[7]. Accompanying fractures of the femoral head or neck also occur. An unrecognised acetabular fragment can prevent reduction or result in instability if the acetabular defect is large. In this patient, the dislocation has been complicated by two fragments detached from the acetabular margin. The fragments are situated superiorly and inferiorly.

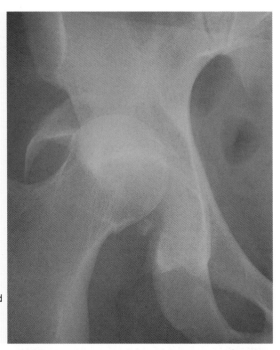

Central dislocation of the head of the femur with fracture of the acetabulum.

The description "central dislocation" is common parlance for this finding. It is not a true dislocation because the femoral head remains within the socket... but it has been forced through the medial wall and lies, in part, within the pelvis.

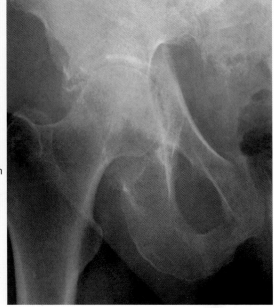

Dislocation following total hip replacement (THR).

Easy to recognise. Occurs much more commonly following a THR for a femoral neck fracture than after an elective THR for other indications[9].

Most dislocations occur in the early postoperative period. Some will dislocate later and attend the Emergency Department; some will become recurrent dislocators.

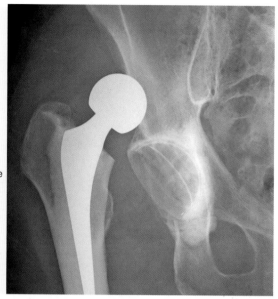

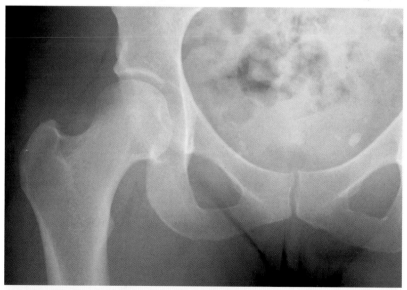

The most basic requirement.

Your ability to detect subtle fractures involving the hip and the adjacent pelvis depends upon your awareness of the normal radiological anatomy (pp. 228–229). Good understanding is essential. This radiograph is normal.

Pitfall

Os acetabuli.

A small bone fragment/ ossicle at the superior margin of the acetabular rim is a common finding. It might represent an unfused secondary ossification centre (an os acetabuli), or a fragment due to femero-acetabular impingement[10].

This ossicle/fragment is most unlikely to represent an acute fracture.

A specialist orthopaedic assessment will invariably distinguish between an unimportant ossicle (an os acetabuli) and an impingement fragment representing a longstanding injury.

See also p. 226.

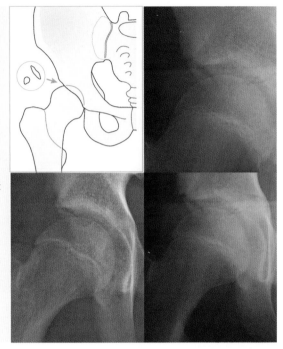

References

1. Parker M, Johansen A. Hip fracture. BMJ 2006; 333: 27–30.
2. Parker MJ. Missed hip fractures. Arch Emerg Med 1992; 9: 23–27.
3. Michaelsson K, Weiderpass E, Farahmand BY et al. Differences in risk factor patterns between cervical and trochanteric hip fractures. Swedish Hip Fracture Study Group. Osteoporos Int 1999; 10: 487–494.
4. Anderson S. Lower extremity injuries in youth sports. Ped Clin North Am 2002; 49: 627–641.
5. Rossi F, Dragoni S. Acute avulsion fractures of the pelvis in adolescent competitive athletes: prevalence, location,and sports distribution of 203 cases collected. Skeletal Radiol 2001; 30: 127–131.
6. Brandser EA, El-Koury GY, Kathol MH. Adolescent hamstring avulsions that simulate tumours. Emerg Radiol 1995; 2: 273–278.
7. Hak DJ, Goulet JA. Severity of injuries associated with traumatic hip dislocation as a result of motor vehicle collisions. J Trauma 1999; 47: 60–63.
8. Clegg TE, Roberts CS, Greene JW, Prather BA. Hip dislocations – Epidemiology, treatment, and outcomes. Injury 2010; 41: 329–334.
9. Gregory RJ, Gibson MJ, Moran CG. Dislocation after primary arthroplasty for subcapital fracture of the hip. Wide range of movement is a risk factor. J Bone Joint Surg Br 1991; 73: 11–12.
10. Martinez AE, Li SM, Ganz R, Beck M. Os acetabuli in femero-acetabular impingement: stress fracture or unfused secondary ossification centre of the acetabular rim? Hip Int 2006; 16: 281–286.

15 Knee

The standard radiographs

AP and **Lateral.**

Suspected patella fracture, but AP & lateral are equivocal: **Skyline view**.

Occasionally, a **Tunnel view** to evaluate the intercondylar area.

Regularly overlooked injuries

- Plateau fracture.
- Segond fracture.
- Small fragments in the joint.
- Vertical fracture of the patella[1].

Abbreviations

ACL, anterior cruciate ligament;
AP, anteroposterior;
FFL, fat–fluid level;
LCL, lateral capsular ligament;
MCL, medial capsular ligament;
PCL, posterior cruciate ligament.

Normal anatomy

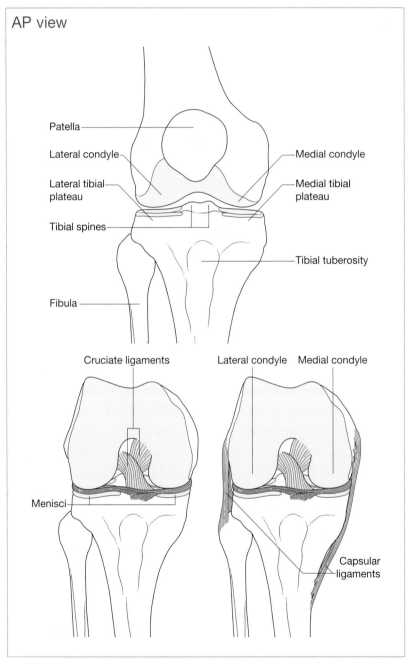

AP view

Patella

Lateral condyle

Lateral tibial plateau

Tibial spines

Fibula

Medial condyle

Medial tibial plateau

Tibial tuberosity

Cruciate ligaments

Menisci

Lateral condyle   Medial condyle

Capsular ligaments

Lateral view

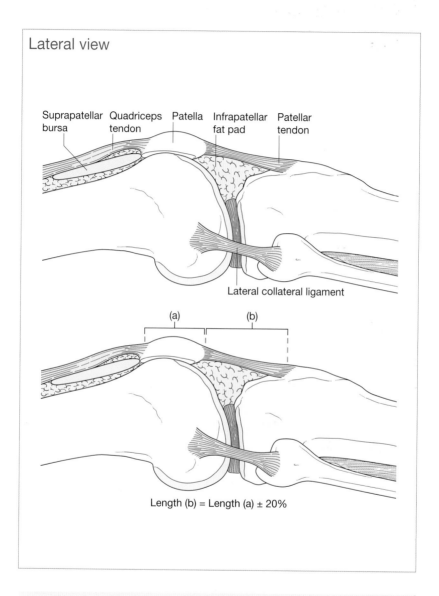

Suprapatellar bursa · Quadriceps tendon · Patella · Infrapatellar fat pad · Patellar tendon

Lateral collateral ligament

(a)   (b)

Length (b) = Length (a) ± 20%

Normal position of the patella—a useful rule:

On the lateral radiograph the distance from the tibial tubercle (on the anterior aspect of the tibia) to the lower pole of the patella should approximate to the length of the patella itself ±20%. This rule is relevant to diagnosing a rupture of the patellar tendon[1–3].

Analysis: the checklists

The AP radiograph

Adults: a five-point checklist

Check:

1. The "intercondylar eminence" (ie the tibial spines) of the tibia and the condylar surfaces of the femur.

2. The head and neck of the fibula.

3. The tibial plateau:

   ☐ Each plateau should be smooth. No steps, no layering, no disruptions.

   ☐ The subchondral bone should not show any focal increase in density.

   ☐ A perpendicular line drawn at the most lateral margin of the femoral condyle should not have more than 5 mm of the lateral margin of the tibial condyle outside of it. A similar rule can be applied to the relationship between the medial femoral condyle and the medial tibial plateau.

4. The patella. Look through the superimposed femur.

5. Finally, check for any small fragments of bone—anywhere at all.

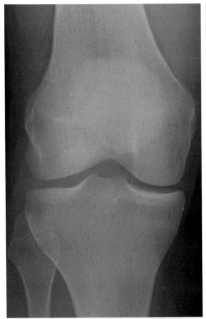

Normal AP.

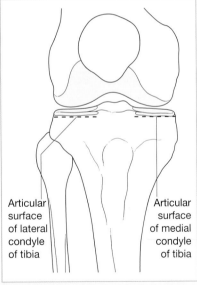

Articular surface of lateral condyle of tibia

Articular surface of medial condyle of tibia

Tibial articular surfaces. Appear as an oval on either side of the intercondylar eminence. These ovals should be smooth without any steps or layering.

In the normal knee a perpendicular line drawn at the most lateral or medial margin of the femur should have no more than 5 mm of adjacent tibia outside of it. If this rule is broken suspect a plateau fracture.

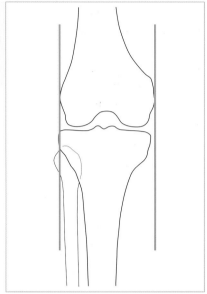

Children: an eight-point checklist

1–5 as for adults, but also check:

6. The growth plates of femur, tibia, and fibula. Is there an epiphyseal fracture? (See pp. 14–17).

7. The cortex of the femur and tibia. Is there a Greenstick or Torus fracture? (See pp. 18–19.)

8. The condylar surfaces of the femur. Is there an osteochondral lesion/fracture? (See pp. 28–29.)

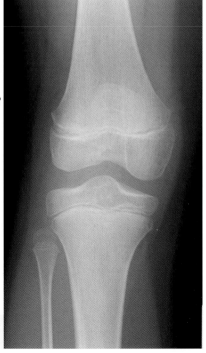

Normal AP.

Knee

The lateral radiograph

It is important to understand the normal and abnormal appearance of the suprapatellar bursa—if abnormal, this often suggests a fracture or ligament damage[4-6].

Adults and children: a six-point checklist

Check:

1. For a joint effusion[4-7]. Present if the **suprapatellar strip** exceeds 5 mm (see below).

2. For a fat–fluid level in the suprapatellar bursa… an intra-articular fracture.

3. The condylar surfaces of the femur. Are they smooth?

4. The patella. Is the articular surface smooth?

5. The position of the patella.

6. For any small fragments of bone—no matter how small.

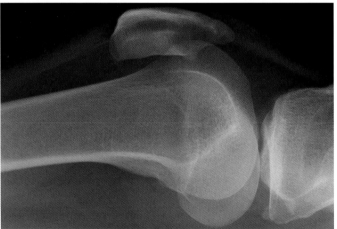

Normal lateral.

A soft tissue band (the **suprapatellar strip**) separates the prefemoral fat pad from the suprapatellar fat pad. Normally its AP width is no more than 5 mm[4,7].

The normal suprapatellar strip is, in effect, an undistended suprapatellar bursa.

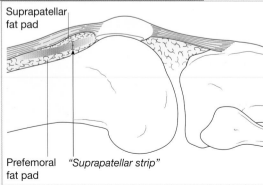

Suprapatellar fat pad

Prefemoral fat pad   *"Suprapatellar strip"*

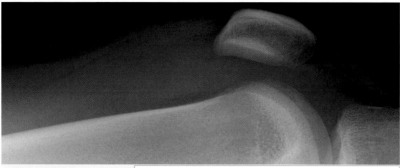

Large effusion.

Note the marked differences compared with the normal appearances on the page opposite.

The suprapatellar strip is markedly widened.

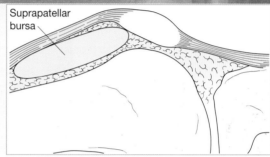

Suprapatellar bursa

Effusion with a fat–fluid level.

In the Emergency Department the lateral view of the knee is obtained with a horizontal X-ray beam (conventionally referred to as a "HBL"). A fat–fluid level occurs when fat (arrowheads) lies on top of blood in the suprapatellar bursa. The fat has been released from bone marrow and consequently the fat–fluid level indicates an intra-articular fracture[7–9].

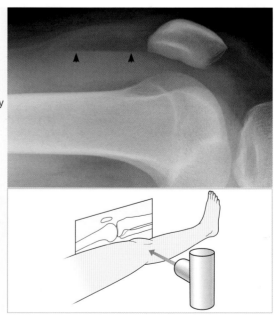

The common fractures

Tibial plateau fracture

Usually seen as a depression in the lateral plateau following violent impaction by the lateral femoral condyle. The so-called 'car bumper' or 'fender' fracture. Many, but by no means all, are true car bumper injuries. Sports injuries and falls at home are other frequent causes.

- Radiographic evidence of an impacted fracture may be subtle. There are four features to look for (see pp. 252–253). Sometimes only one or two will be present.

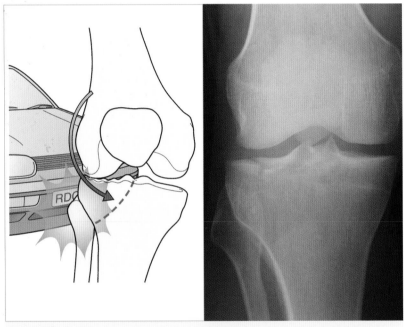

80% of tibial plateau fractures involve the lateral plateau as a result of a severe valgus stress combined with a violent compressive force which drives the femoral condyle into the tibial plateau.

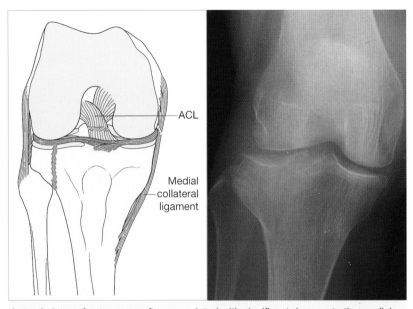

Lateral plateau fractures are often associated with significant damage to the medial collateral ligament or to a cruciate ligament.

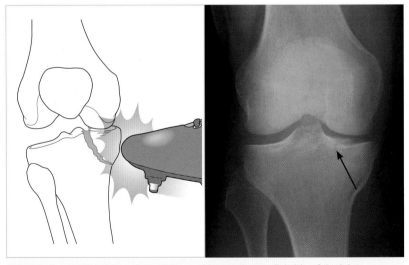

Injury to the medial plateau (arrow) from a blow to the medial side of the joint.

251

Tibial plateau fracture—the four features to look for

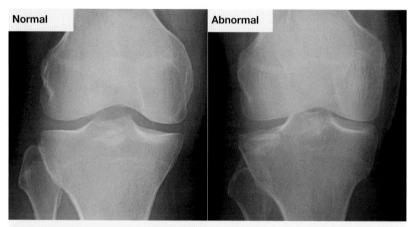

Feature (1). The normal plateau is smooth—but this alters when the plateau is fractured. The fractured plateau has an irregular surface or becomes layered. Additionally, fracture lines may extend inferiorly.

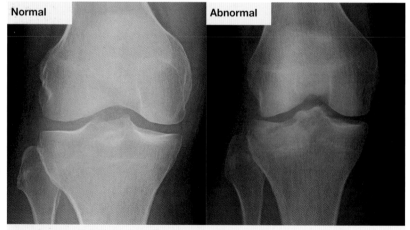

Feature (2). An area of focal increase in density below the plateau due to bone compression causing an impaction. Lateral plateau fracture.

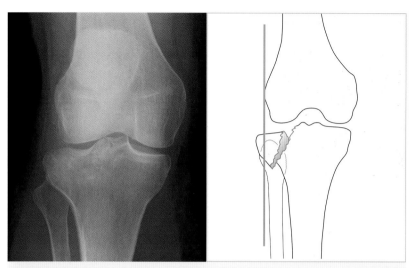

Feature (3). Tibial margin displacement. Use this rule: "a perpendicular line drawn at the most lateral margin of the femur should not have more than 5 mm of the adjacent margin of the tibia beyond it". Lateral plateau fracture.

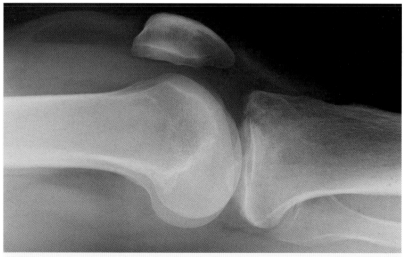

Feature (4). On the lateral radiograph, in most cases of a fracture involving a plateau there will be a fat–fluid level[8,9], as shown here.

Fracture through the body of the patella

Usually caused by a direct blow. Vertical, horizontal and comminuted fractures occur. A violent contraction of the quadriceps can cause a transverse fracture in an athlete.

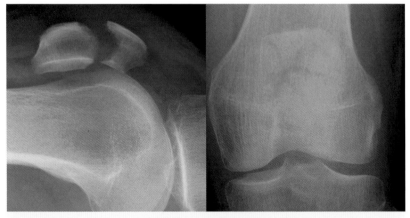

Horizontal (left) and comminuted (right) fractures of the patella.

Caution: this fracture was not seen on the standard views of the knee. Occasionally this occurs, usually with an undisplaced vertical fracture. Clinical concern will determine whether an additional projection is necessary[1,7].

This is a skyline view.

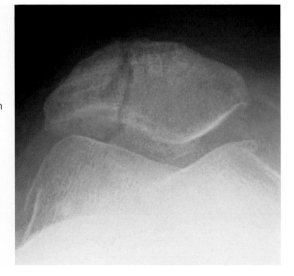

Osteochondral fracture: articular surface of the patella

Often consequent on high energy trauma in young patients. Articular surfaces shear against each other. The medial surface of the patella is usually affected.

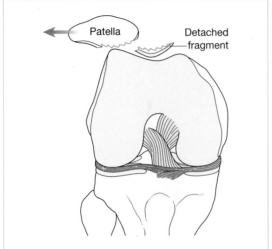

Shearing force as shown.

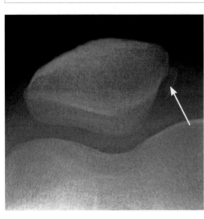

Sometimes the defect in the articular surface, or a detached fragment (arrow), is only shown on a skyline (ie tangential) view[1,10].

Occasionally a shearing injury to the articular surface of the lateral femoral condyle occurs at the time of a transient dislocation of the patella. This can cause a visible defect in the femur and/or a small sliver of bone within the joint.

Neck of fibula fracture

Don't dismiss an isolated fracture too lightly. These fractures of the fibula are often consequent on high energy trauma. Damage to the collateral or cruciate ligaments within the joint are well recognised associations.

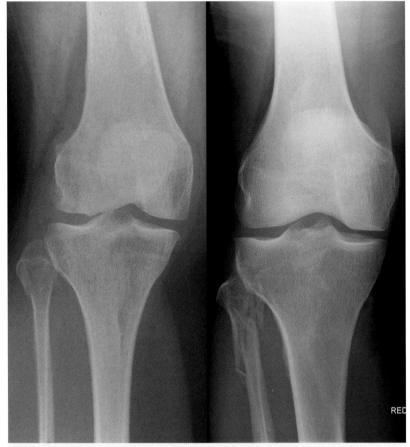

Both of these patients show a fracture through the neck of the fibula.
In addition, each patient had also sustained a severe ligamentous injury.

Osteochondritis dissecans of the knee

Repetitive trauma may cause a defect in the articular surface of the femur. Most commonly affecting the lateral aspect of the medial femoral condyle. See pp. 28–29.

Supracondylar and intracondylar fractures of the femur

Most commonly consequent on high energy trauma in the young; typically a road traffic accident. These fractures also occur in elderly patients with severe osteoporosis who have fallen. Detecting the fracture on the radiographs is straightforward.

Fracture/avulsion of the tibial spine

An avulsion fracture of the tibial spine (the intercondylar eminence) indicates a cruciate ligament injury because this area is the site of attachment of these ligaments.

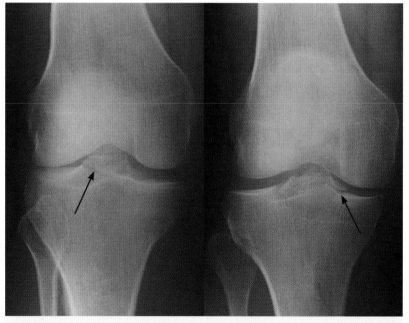

Avulsion fractures (arrows) of the tibial spine.

Small fragments around the knee

Any small fragment is important. It will warn you that an important soft tissue injury is likely.

Cruciate ligament injury[11,12]

The cruciate ligaments insert into the intercondylar region (ie anteriorly and posteriorly) of the tibial plateau. A rupture may be accompanied by avulsion of a small fragment detached from the site of the ligament's insertion into the tibia.

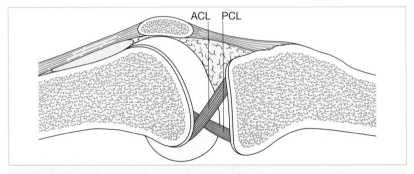

ACL   PCL

Insertion of the ACL and PCL, shown on this intercondylar sagittal section.

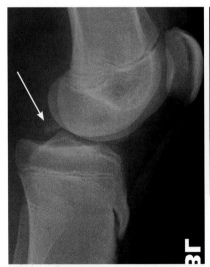

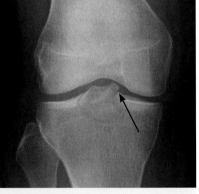

ACL avulsion fracture.

If a tiny fragment of bone (arrow) is identified close to the intercondylar eminence (ie the tibial spine) this is invariably consequent on an avulsion of the tibial attachment of the anterior cruciate ligament. Occasionally, the detached bone fragment may be lying loose and visible elsewhere within the joint.

PCL avulsion fracture.

If a tiny fragment (arrow) is identified close to the tibial articular surface posteriorly then the PCL is likely to have been injured.

Cruciate ligament or meniscus injury— Segond fracture[11–14]

A tear of the lateral capsular ligament may cause a cortical avulsion where it is attached to the tibia. The tear is consequent on forceful internal rotation and varus stress. This cortical avulsion is termed a Segond fracture.

A Segond fracture has a strong association with a tear of the anterior cruciate ligament (ACL) and/or a meniscal injury. More than 75% of patients with a Segond fracture have torn the ACL.

A Segond fracture is regarded as the most frequent indirect sign of an ACL tear seen on a plain radiograph.

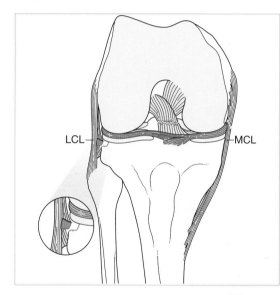

The lateral capsular ligament has pulled a fragment away from the cortex of the tibia. This detached fragment represents the Segond fracture.

Some of the possible associated ligamentous tears are illustrated.

LCL = lateral capsular ligament.

MCL = medial capsular ligament.

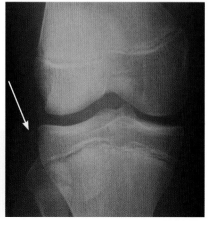

Segond fracture. The fracture fragment (arrow) lies at the margin of the lateral tibial plateau just below the joint line.

The avulsed fragment may be very tiny. Size varies from 1 mm to 27 mm[14].

259

A common dislocation

Patella dislocation[15,16]

The knee joint is most vulnerable when the leg is extended. It is then that the patella is least stable and most vulnerable to an external force.

Fracture complication: in approximately 20% of patients who have dislocated the patella there will be a small sliver of bone detectable on the plain radiographs. This fragment detaches from the patella or from the lateral femoral articular surface as part of a shearing injury during the dislocation.

With many patients, who have suffered a transient patella dislocation and subsequently attend the Emergency Department, the dislocation will already have reduced spontaneously. In these patients it is wise to obtain a patellar view (skyline view) as well as the standard knee radiographs as this will increase the chances of detecting a fragment that might have sheared off at the time of dislocation.

Infrequent but important injuries

Epiphyseal growth plate fractures.

See pp. 14–15.

Maisonneuve fracture.

Fracture through the proximal fibula, and an associated ankle fracture. See p. 284.

Stress fracture of the tibia.

The most common site for a stress fracture around the knee is in the proximal tibia (arrows).

The stress fracture in this patient is fairly typical— it appears as a sclerotic band.

Sometimes the band is accompanied by periosteal new bone along the adjacent cortical margin.

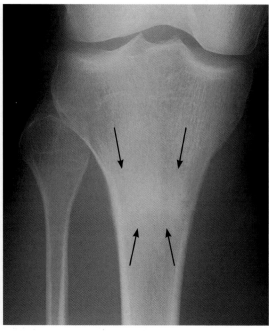

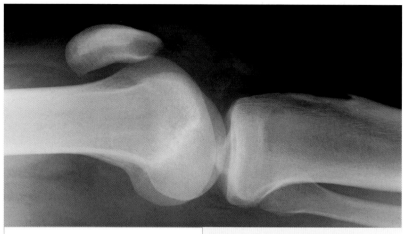

Rupture of the patellar tendon.

Most commonly the result of direct trauma. The rupture is through the proximal part of the tendon close to the inferior pole of the patella.

Identified on the lateral radiograph by a high position of the patella (as above).

A high position? Apply this rule: in the normal knee, the distance from the tibial tubercle to the lower pole of the patella should not exceed the length of the patella by more than 20% (see below).

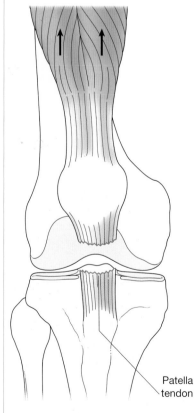

Patella tendon

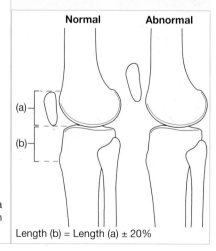

	Normal	Abnormal
(a)		
(b)		

Length (b) = Length (a) ± 20%

Pitfalls

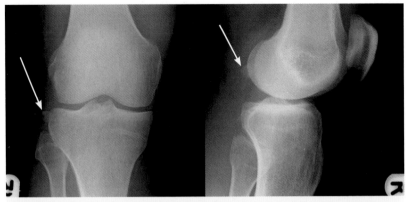

The fabella. A common sesamoid bone in the tendon of the lateral head of the gastrocnemius muscle. Its posterior position is characteristic. Do not confuse the fabella (arrow) with a fracture fragment or a loose body.

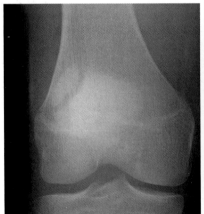

Bipartite patella. The patella may develop from several ossification centres, which sometimes remain unfused in the adult. Two unfused centres are most common. The smaller centre is characteristically positioned in the upper outer quadrant, and may mimic a fracture. An ossification centre will have a well defined sclerotic (corticated) edge and its margin will match the contour of the adjacent bone. Occasionally there are three unfused centres (tripartite patella).

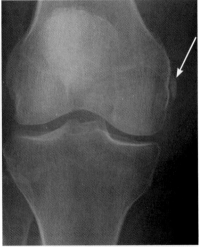

Pellegrini–Stieda lesion. Calcification (arrow) adjacent to the medial epicondyle following a previous sprain of the medial collateral ligament. Do not mistake this lesion for a fracture fragment.

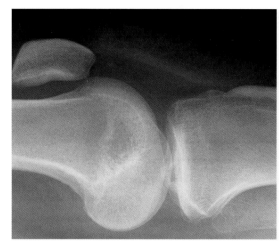

Patella Alta.

A high patella position due to a developmental elongation of the infrapatellar tendon. Do not confuse with a patella tendon rupture. A Patella Alta predisposes to patella subluxation.

A rough guide: *"if the inferior pole of the patella is situated entirely above the intercondylar notch of the femur then this is consistent with a Patella Alta"*.

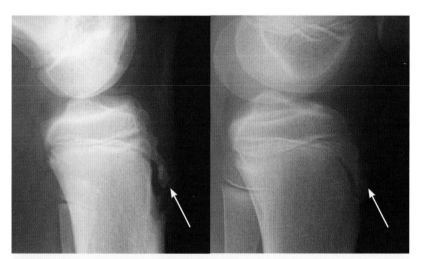

The tibial tubercle and Osgood–Schlatter's disease

Osgood-Schlatter's disease is a condition that occurs most commonly in adolescent boys. It is suspected to be a chronic avulsion injury resulting from recurrent episodes of minor trauma[11,17].

A plain film diagnosis cannot be made with absolute certainty because the normal ossification centre can appear very fragmented, irregular, or separate. This diagnosis is best made on clinical history and examination.

Do not misinterpret a normal appearance. The two examples shown here (arrows) are normal.

References

1. Capps GW, Hayes CW. Easily missed injuries around the knee. Radiographics 1994; 14: 1191–1210.
2. Insall J, Salvati E. Patella position in the normal knee joint. Radiology 1971; 101: 101–104.
3. Newberg A, Wales L. Radiographic diagnosis of quadriceps tendon rupture. Radiology 1977; 125: 367–371.
4. Hall FM. Radiographic diagnosis and accuracy in knee joint effusions. Radiology 1975; 115: 49–54.
5. Butt WP, Lederman H, Chuang S. Radiology of the suprapatellar region. Clin Rad 1983; 34: 511–522.
6. Fishwick NG, Learmouth DJ, Finlay DB. Knee effusions, radiology and acute knee trauma. Br J Radiol 1994; 67: 934–937.
7. The Knee. Chan O. (ed). ABC of Emergency Radiology. 3rd ed. Wiley Blackwell, 2013.
8. Ferguson J, Knottenbelt JD. Lipohaemarthrosis in knee trauma; an experience of 907 cases. Injury 1994; 25: 311–312.
9. Lee JH, Weissman BN, Nikpoor N et al. Lipohemarthrosis of the knee: a review of recent experiences. Radiology 1989; 173: 189–191.
10. Rorabeck CH, Bobechko WP. Acute dislocation of the patella with osteochondral fracture: a review of eighteen cases. J Bone Joint Surg 1976; 58: 237–240.
11. Gottsegen C , Eyer B, White E et al. Avulsion Fractures of the Knee: Imaging Findings and Clinical Significance. RadioGraphics 2008; 28: 1755–1770.
12. Delzell PB, Schils JP, Recht MP. Subtle fractures about the knee: innocuous-appearing yet indicative of significant internal derangement Am J Roentgenol 1996; 167: 699–703.
13. Sferopoulos NK, Rafailidis D, Traios S, Christoforides J. Avulsion fractures of the lateral tibial condyle in children. Injury 2006; 37: 57–60.
14. Goldman AB, Pavlov H, Rubenstein D. The Segond fracture of the proximal tibia: a small avulsion that reflects major ligamentous damage. Am J Roentgenol 1988; 151: 1163–1167.
15. Haas JP, Collins MS and Stuart MJ. The "sliver sign": a specific radiographic sign of acute lateral patellar dislocation. Skeletal Radiol 2012; 41: 595–601.
16. Anderson S. Lower extremity injuries in youth sports. Pediatr Clin North Am 2002; 49: 627–641.
17. Rosenberg ZS, Kawelblum M, Cheung YY et al. Osgood–Schlatter lesion: fracture or tendinitis? Scintigraphic, CT, and MR imaging features. Radiology 1992; 185: 853–858.

16 Ankle & hindfoot

Regularly overlooked injuries[1]

Talus: talar dome osteochondral lesion; neck of talus fracture; medial or lateral process fractures. **Calcaneum**: acute fracture; stress fracture.

Syndesmotic widening (tear of tibiofibular membrane).

Base of 5th metatarsal fracture.

The standard radiographs

Ankle: **AP mortice** (20° internal rotation) and **Lateral**. Sometimes a **Straight AP**[2].

Calcaneal injury: an additional **Axial**.

Abbreviations

AP, anterior-posterior; AVN, avascular necrosis; CT, computed tomography; MT, metatarsal; RTA, road traffic accident.

Normal anatomy

Lateral view—bones and joints

The lateral and medial malleoli can be identified. Helpful hints to aid identification:

- The lateral malleolus extends more inferiorly than the medial malleolus.
- The medial malleolus has a notch inferiorly.

The posterior lip (or tubercle) of the tibia, conventionally and inaccurately referred to as the posterior malleolus, is well shown.

The calcaneum and its sustentaculum tali are demonstrated. Bohler's angle can be assessed for normality.

The base of the 5th metatarsal is often included.

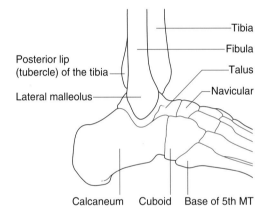

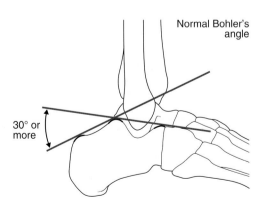

Lateral view—ligaments

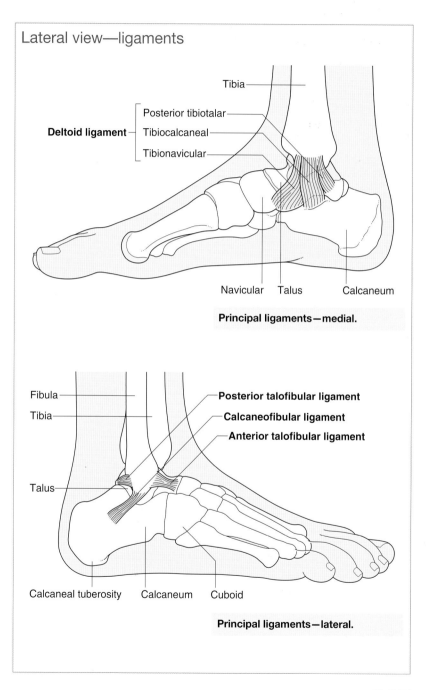

Tibia

Deltoid ligament — Posterior tibiotalar —
Tibiocalcaneal —
Tibionavicular —

Navicular   Talus   Calcaneum

Principal ligaments—medial.

Fibula —
Tibia —

Posterior talofibular ligament
Calcaneofibular ligament
Anterior talofibular ligament

Talus —

Calcaneal tuberosity   Calcaneum   Cuboid

Principal ligaments—lateral.

AP mortice

The mortice projection is obtained with slight (20°) internal rotation so that the fibula does not overlap the talus.

The joint space should be of uniform width all the way around. This space is well seen medially, it continues over the superior aspect of the dome of the talus, on to the lateral side of the joint.

The width of the joint space measures approximately 4 mm^2.

The surface of the talar dome should be smooth, smooth, smooth. No irregularity, no notching, no defect.

The lateral process (also known as the lateral tubercle) of the talus is an important structure. The talocalcaneal ligament attaches to this part of the bone.

A useful rule: the bones of the tibia and fibula should always overlap on the mortice view. Any clear separation between these two bones should lead you to question whether the interosseous membrane is torn.

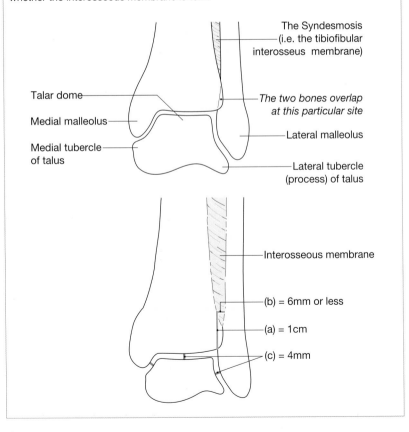

Axial projection—calcaneum

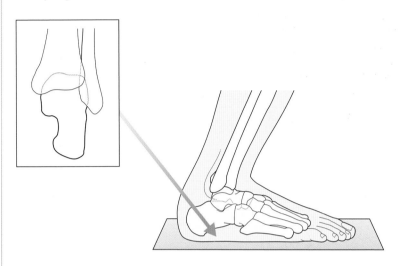

The posterior two thirds of the bone is well shown; the anteriorly positioned sustentaculum tali is often not as well visualised on the radiograph.

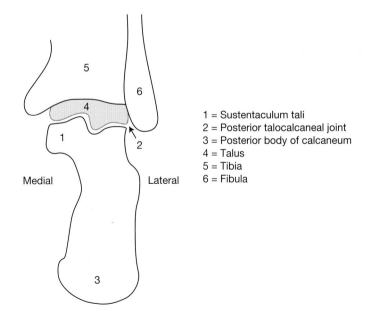

1 = Sustentaculum tali
2 = Posterior talocalcaneal joint
3 = Posterior body of calcaneum
4 = Talus
5 = Tibia
6 = Fibula

269

Analysis: the checklists[1,3,4]

AP mortice

Check the:

- Malleoli—fracture or... fractures?

- Tibiofibular interosseous membrane—any suggestion of a rupture?

  - If normal, the tibia and fibula should show some degree of overlap.

  - A measurement: the width of the space between the distal tibia and fibula at a point 1.0 cm proximal to the tibial articular surface should not exceed 6 mm[5].

- Talus

  - Dome—smooth?

  - Medial and lateral processes (ie the tubercles, p. 268)—any fragmentation?

- Joint width—does any part exceed the normal 4 mm[3]?

- Epiphyses and growth plates in children—normal? (see pp. 15 and 280).

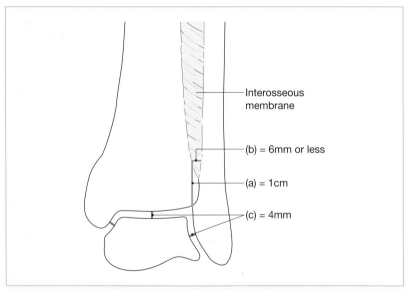

Normal features and measurements (ie rules of thumb) relating to:
(1) the interosseous membrane, and (2) the various articulations at the mortice joint.

Normal AP mortice view.

All of the checkpoints are normal.

Note that part of the fibula overlaps part of the tibia. This is a characteristically normal appearance on a mortice view.

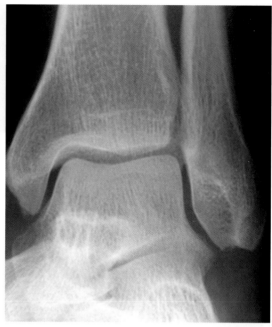

Normal AP mortice view. A child.

The growth plates and all of the other checkpoints are normal.

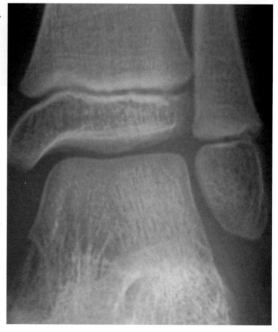

Lateral view

Check the:

- Tibia
  - ☐ Cortices—intact?
  - ☐ Articular surface—smooth?
- Fibula
  - ☐ Oblique fracture line?
- Talus
  - ☐ Neck—intact?
  - ☐ Articulation with the navicular bone —can you see a normal joint?
- Calcaneum
  - ☐ Any fracture lines?
  - ☐ Bohler's angle—normal?
  - ☐ Anterior process—normal?
- 5th metatarsal
  - ☐ Fracture of the base?

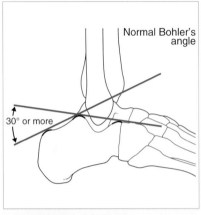

Measuring Bohler's angle.

Draw a line from the highest point anteriorly to the highest midpoint. Then draw a line from the highest point posteriorly to the highest midpoint. The angle subtended should be 30° or more.

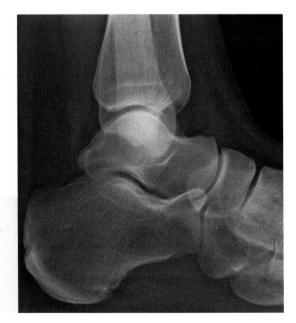

Normal lateral.

Checkpoints: all normal.

Joints: all normal.

Bohler's angle: normal.

Base of 5th metatarsal: normal.

Axial view

Check the:

- Calcaneum.
    - Any fracture lines?
    - Cortices—intact?

The normal standing foot seen from behind. This drawing may help you to understand the anatomy on the axial view of the calcaneum. The sustentaculum tali is the shelf-like part of the calcaneum which extends medially to support part of the head of the talus.

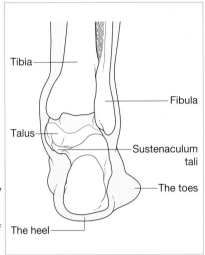

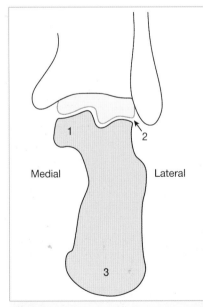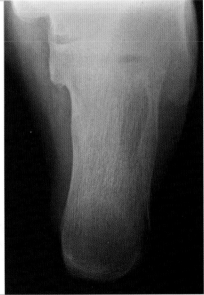

Normal axial view.

1 = Sustentaculum tali
2 = Posterior talocalcaneal joint
3 = Posterior body of calcaneum

Common fractures/torn ligaments

The malleoli[3,6]

- Most ankle fractures involve one or both malleoli. These fractures are often easy to diagnose because you will know precisely which bones are tender.

- The direction of the applied forces will determine the particular fracture (or fractures) and any associated ligamentous damage:

    - In (a) below, abduction and external rotation forces.

    - In (b) below, adduction forces.

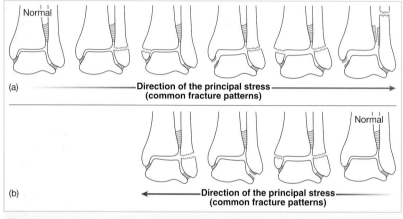

(a) ←——— **Direction of the principal stress** ———→
(common fracture patterns)

(b) ←——— **Direction of the principal stress** ———
(common fracture patterns)

This illustration is adapted in modified form from *Tidy's Physiotherapy*[7].

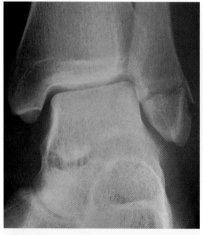

Transverse fracture of the lateral malleolus.

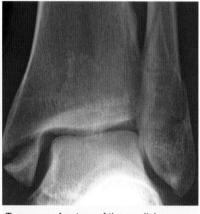

Transverse fracture of the medial malleolus; oblique and transverse fractures of the distal fibula and lateral malleolus; lateral subluxation of talus.

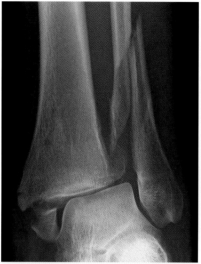

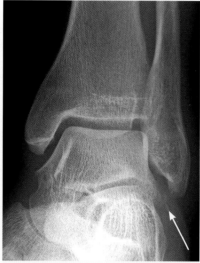

Multiple fractures affect the tibia and fibula. Note the wide separation at the tibiofibular joint indicating rupture of the interosseous membrane.

Small fragments (arrow) are detached from the lateral process of the talus.

This indicates ligamentous damage.

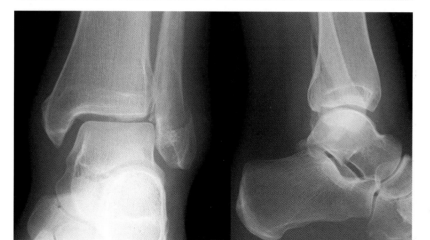

We have taken illustrative license with the earlier cases in this section by only providing AP radiographs. In all instances it is essential to assess both the AP and lateral radiographs as a pair. In this patient the AP view shows the transverse fracture of the lateral malleolus and the lateral subluxation of the talus. The lateral view shows the full extent of the fibular fracture and its displacement. It also allows assessment of the posterior lip of the tibia, the talus and the calcaneum.

Base of the 5th metatarsal

An avulsion fracture. This common injury results from avulsion of the metatarsal tuberosity at the insertion of the peroneus brevis tendon. The fracture occurs as a consequence of forced inversion.

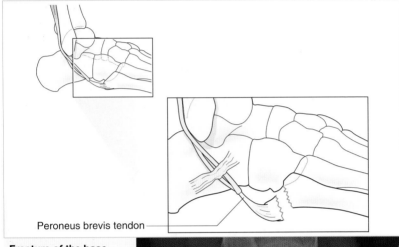

Peroneus brevis tendon

Fracture of the base of the 5th metatarsal.

A twisted ankle (ie if a forced inversion injury) will often result in a transverse fracture of the base of the 5th metatarsal. The radiograph shows a typical appearance.

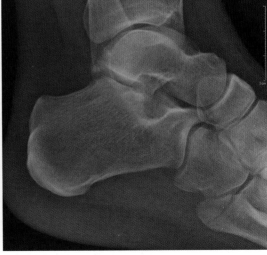

The calcaneum

The calcaneum is the most commonly injured bone of the hindfoot. Types of calcaneal fracture are shown on pp. 278–279. See also infrequent calcaneal injuries on p. 288.

Most severe injuries occur following a fall from a height.

The fracture partly results from the talus driving into the calcaneum, like a wedge of steel slamming down into a block of wood.

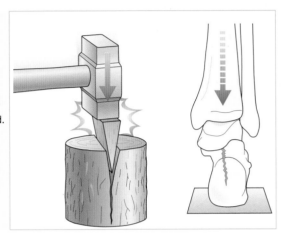

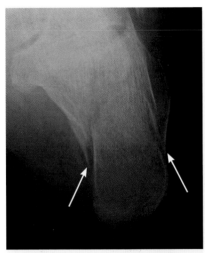

If a calcaneal fracture is suspected then an axial view should be obtained.

The fractures (arrows) through the body of the calcaneum are well shown.

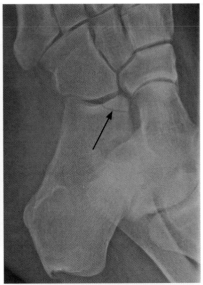

Some fractures, particularly those involving the anterior process of the calcaneum (arrow), can result from a simple twisting injury.

277

Several types of calcaneal fracture

Intra-articular (75%)

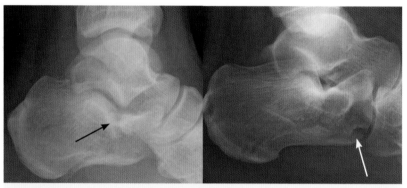

Intra-articular fractures (arrows) involve the subtalar joint (left) or calcaneo-cuboid joint (right).

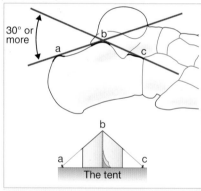

30° or more

b

a

c

b

a   c

The tent

a

b

c

Collapsed tent

Some fractures will only become apparent when Bohler's angle is assessed on the lateral view (above).

This angle is normally 30–40°. If the fracture results in flattening of the bone then the angle will be considerably less than 30° (above right).

Flattening of Bohler's angle is the dominant feature in the calcaneal fracture shown in the radiograph on the right.

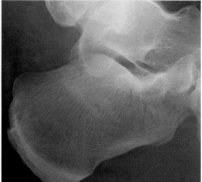

Extra-articular (25%)

Usually more difficult to detect compared with intra-articular fractures.

Extra-articular fractures involve the posterior part of the calcaneum or, alternatively, the anterior process of the bone[1,4,8]. Most of these fractures are sustained following a fall on the heel, but not from a great height. Occasionally a twisting injury may be the cause.

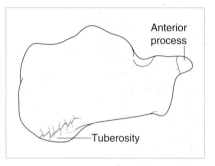

A sclerotic line or density in the body of the calcaneum (arrow) may be the only evidence of an impacted fracture. This is an extra-articular fracture through the tuberosity of the calcaneum and was sustained during a relatively minor fall on to the heel.

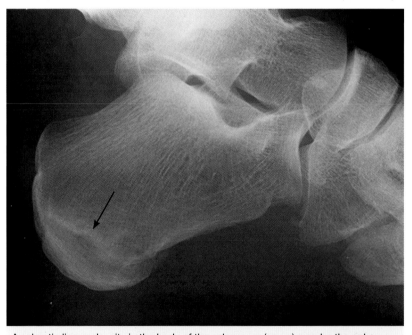

Growth plate (Salter–Harris) fractures

- Relatively common in children. A distal growth plate injury of the tibia is second in frequency to an injury of the distal growth plate of the radius.

- Growth plate fractures are described in detail on pp. 14–17.

- The most common growth plate fractures (types 1–4) are shown below.

The Salter–Harris classification/description of the fractures that involve the growth plate.

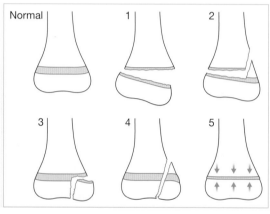

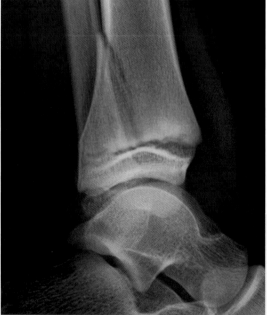

Salter–Harris type 2 fracture of the tibia.

A type 2 fracture is the most commonly occurring of the fractures that involve the growth plate.

Ligamentous injuries

Torn medial or lateral ligaments

If there is widening of one side of the mortice joint space then there is commonly an associated fracture elsewhere. Suspect widening if the joint space is wider than 4 mm medially or laterally[3]. **Caution:** the radiographs may appear normal even when there is severe ligamentous damage. Sometimes stress views will be required.

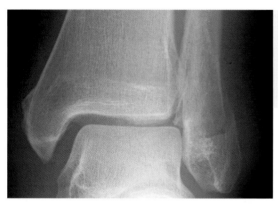

Fracture of the fibula.

The widened medial joint space indicates an associated ligamentous tear/rupture (the deltoid ligament).

Tear of the interosseous membrane

This injury is very easy to overlook[1,5,9,10]. The AP radiograph will often provide evidence of a tear/rupture. Look for widening of the space between the distal tibia and the fibula. A useful rule of thumb: suspect a tear of the tough tibiofibular syndesmosis whenever the distal tibia and fibula do not overlap slightly on the AP mortice view.
Also… apply the 6 mm rule (see p. 270).

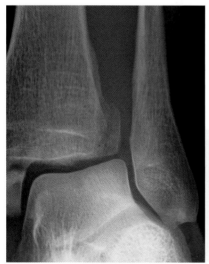

The wide separation between the tibia and the fibula indicates a major tear of the interosseous membrane (the syndesmosis).

This membrane is a fairly rigid structure. It holds the shafts of the tibia and fibula together, and extends downwards from the superior to the inferior tibiofibular joint.

Infrequent but important injuries

Fractures of the talus

Talar fractures are rare. Many result from a high energy injury, often a road traffic accident or a fall from a height.

Body of the talus[4,11]

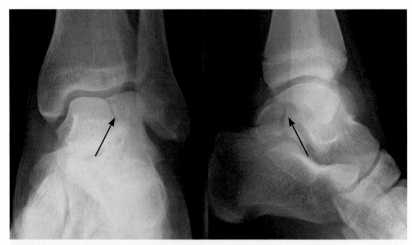

Fractures (arrows) can occur in the coronal, sagittal or horizontal planes.

Neck of the talus[4,11]

An important injury because of the high risk of subsequent avascular necrosis (AVN) and secondary degenerative arthritis. AVN is caused by disruption of the blood supply to the body of the talus. Displacement of the fracture increases the probability of AVN. A displaced fracture is easy to detect. An undisplaced fracture is easy to overlook.

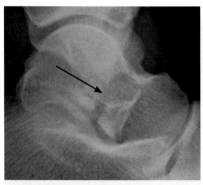
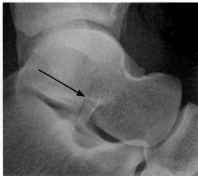

Displaced fracture through the neck of the talus (arrow).

Undisplaced fracture through the neck of the talus (arrow).

Talar dome–osteochondral fracture

A small but clinically important impaction fracture, usually consequent on an inversion injury[1,12]. The term osteochondritis dissecans was used in early descriptions of this lesion when it was assumed that the pathology was a spontaneous necrosis of bone in the dome of the talus. It is now generally accepted that most of these lesions are actually osteochondral fractures resulting from trauma.

In many cases the talar lesion is not an acute injury but has resulted from an earlier shearing or compression force.

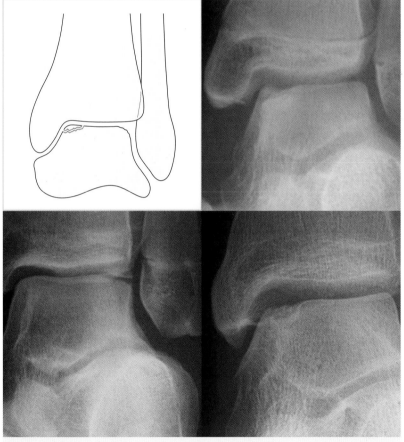

An osteochondral fracture is identified as either a focal defect (ie a lucent area) or an irregularity of the cortex. Most frequently situated on the medial or lateral aspect of the talar dome. Sometimes a small fragment will be detached from the dome and lie free within the joint.

Maisonneuve fracture

The ankle joint is in effect a bone ring and this particular ring extends as high as the knee because of the strong tibiofibular interosseous membrane. On occasion an external rotation injury of the ankle may cause an ankle injury but in addition the forces/energy acting within the interosseous membrane (the tibiofibular syndesmosis) may extend to the upper leg and cause a fracture of the proximal fibula[13]. The high fibular fracture may be overlooked because the main symptoms are around the ankle joint.

This combination injury is known as a Maisonneuve fracture. Suspect this injury whenever clinical examination of the upper leg is painful.

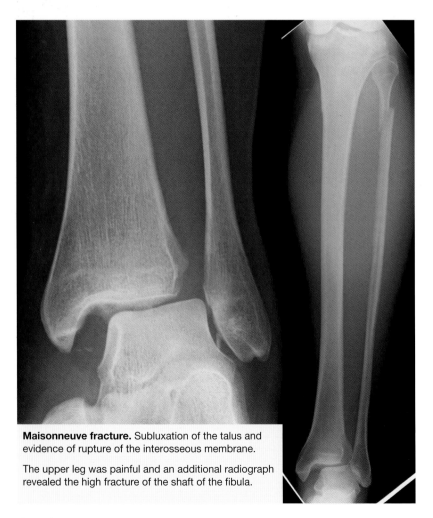

Maisonneuve fracture. Subluxation of the talus and evidence of rupture of the interosseous membrane.

The upper leg was painful and an additional radiograph revealed the high fracture of the shaft of the fibula.

Distal tibial fractures involving the articular surface

These fractures are rare, accounting for less than 1% of fractures of the lower limb[14].

The usual cause: a high energy fall or RTA producing a compression fracture, often with comminution. Compression fractures of the tibia are rare because it is usually the calcaneum that received and accepts the major vertical force and is fractured.

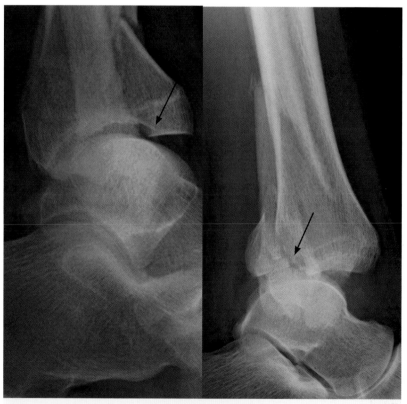

Both patients had fallen from a height. Comminuted fracture of the tibia with involvement of the articular surface (arrows).

Complex Salter–Harris fractures

These two fractures are rare but need to be recognised early, as accurate reduction is essential in order to ensure normal growth and to avoid subsequent ankle deformity.

Triplane fracture[3,15,16]

This Salter–Harris type 4 fracture is a complex multi-directional fracture of the tibial epiphysis. It is a three plane fracture. As follows:

- Sagittal plane: vertical fracture through the epiphysis.

- Horizontal plane: transverse fracture through the growth plate.

- Coronal plane: vertical fracture through the metaphysis.

Always suspect this complex fracture whenever the AP view shows a vertical fracture through the tibial epiphysis. Suspicion necessitates CT for full evaluation.

Pitfall: the full extent of the injury is often not evident on plain radiography.

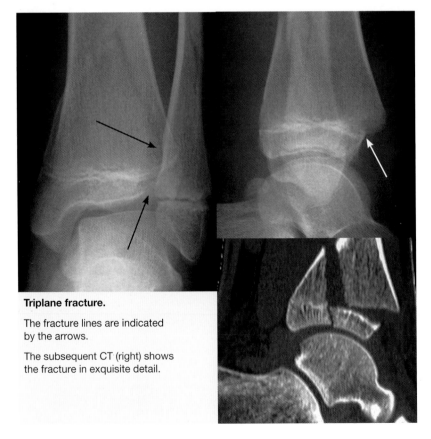

Triplane fracture.

The fracture lines are indicated by the arrows.

The subsequent CT (right) shows the fracture in exquisite detail.

Tillaux fracture[3,16]

This Salter–Harris type 3 fracture is an avulsion fracture through the tibial epiphysis. The fracture involves a partially closed epiphysis (age 11–15 years). It occurs in adolescents in whom the medial part of the growth plate has fused, but the normal fusion has not yet reached the lateral aspect. It is a two plane fracture. As follows:

▨ Vertical plane: through the epiphysis.

▨ Horizontal plane: through the lateral part of the growth plate.

Pitfall. This fracture can sometimes be confused with a Triplane fracture on plain radiography. CT will distinguish.

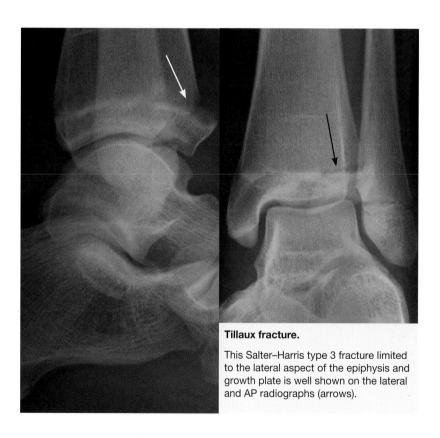

Tillaux fracture.

This Salter–Harris type 3 fracture limited to the lateral aspect of the epiphysis and growth plate is well shown on the lateral and AP radiographs (arrows).

Infrequent calcaneal fractures

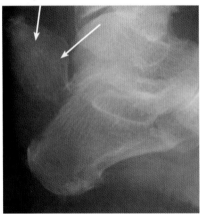 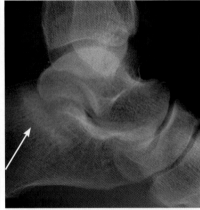

Avulsion fracture of the calcaneal tuberosity (arrows). It represents an avulsion of the Achilles tendon with part of the calcaneum. Occurs most commonly in an elderly patient with severe osteoporosis.

Fatigue fractures due to repetitive stress are rare but do occur. Usually identified as an area of bone sclerosis on the lateral radiograph (arrow).

Os trigonum fracture[17]

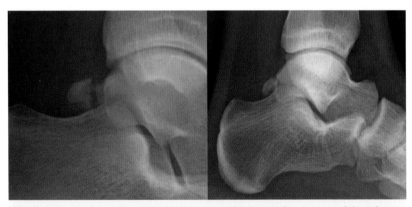

The os trigonum is an elongation/enlargement of the posterior process of the talus. It is present in approximately 50% of feet and can be fused to the posterior aspect of the talus or it can be a free bone on its own. A fracture of a fused os trigonum can occur during a twisting injury at the ankle joint. A very high index of clinical suspicion is essential in order to raise the suggestion of a fracture. The two examples shown here are normal.

Talar dislocations—Infrequent but important

The subtalar joint has two parts and either part can dislocate as a result of a high energy force.

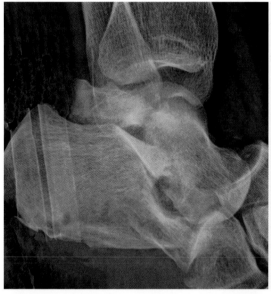

Dislocation of the talocalcaneal joint.

The talonavicular and talocalcaneal articulations are not anatomical—compare this with the normal articulations on the opposite page.

Several fractures/fracture fragments are also present.

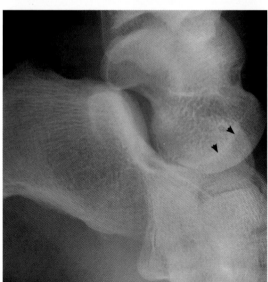

Dislocation of the talonavicular joint.

Note that the head of the talus overlaps, ie it is displaced anterior to, the articular surface of the navicular bone (arrowheads).

The normal appearance at the talonavicular joint is shown in the other figures on the page opposite.

Pitfalls

Calcaneum: the apophysis

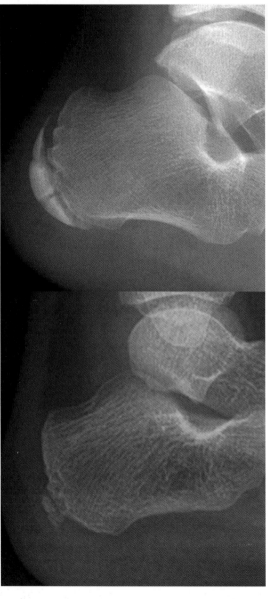

The normal calcaneal apophysis can appear very irregular, fragmented and/or sclerotic, as in these two examples.

Calcaneum: the anterior process

A fracture of the anterior process (p. 279) is a common injury. However, the anterior process can develop from a secondary ossification centre. If this centre does not unite with the parent bone it (the os secundum) can be mistaken for a fracture. Distinguishing between a fracture and an os secundum will depend on correlation with the clinical findings.

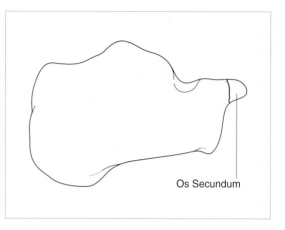

Os Secundum

Normal accessory ossicles

Small bones lying adjacent to the tips of the medial and lateral malleoli are very common. They may be misread as avulsed fracture fragments. Occasionally an ossicle will be difficult to distinguish from a fracture and clinical correlation is important. Fractures are tender, accessory ossicles are not. Also:

- An accessory ossicle has a well defined (ie corticated) outline.

- An acute fracture fragment is ill defined (ie not corticated) on one of its sides.

Normal accessory ossicles at tips of the medial and lateral malleoli in a 10 year old.

A frequent finding.

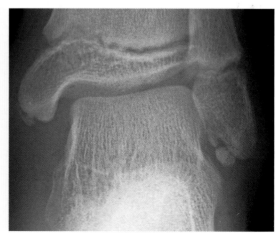

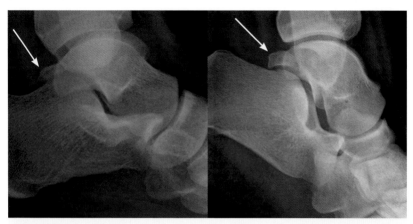

The os trigonum (arrows). A common normal variant (p. 288). It may be attached to, or separate from the talus.

References

1. Brandser EA, Braksiek RJ, El-Khoury GY et al. Missed fractures on emergency room ankle radiographs: an analysis of 433 patients. Emergency Radiology 1997; 4: 295–302.
2. Brandser EA, Berbaum KS, Dorfman DD et al. Contribution of Individual Projections Alone and in Combination for Radiographic Detection of Ankle Fractures. Am J Roentgenol 2000; 174: 1691–1697.
3. Daffner RH. Ankle Trauma. Semin Roentgenol 1994; 29: 134–151.
4. Prokuski LJ, Saltzman CL. Challenging fractures of the foot and ankle. Rad Clin North Am 1997; 35: 655–670.
5. Harper MC, Keller TS. A radiographic evaluation of the tibiofibular syndesmosis. Foot Ankle 1989; 10: 156–160.
6. Hamblen DL, Simpson HR. Adams's Outline of Fractures including joint injuries.12th edn. Churchill Livingstone, 2007.
7. Tidy's Physiotherapy. Porter S (ed.) 15th edn. Churchill Livingstone, Elsevier, 2013.
8. Slatis P, Kiviluoto O, Santavirta S, Laasonen EM. Fractures of the calcaneum. J Trauma 1979; 19: 939–943.
9. Ramsey PL, Hamilton W. Changes in tibiotalar area of contact caused by lateral talar shift. J Bone Joint Surg Am 1976; 58: 356–357.
10. Edwards GS, Delee JC. Ankle diastasis without fracture. Foot Ankle 1984; 4: 305–312.
11. Rammelt S, Zwipp H. Talar neck and body fractures. Injury 2009; 40: 120–135.
12. Canale ST, Belding RH. Osteochondral lesions of the talus. J Bone Joint Surg Am 1980; 62: 97–102.
13. Anderson S. Lower extremity injuries in youth sports. Pediatr Clin North Am 2002; 49: 627–641.
14. Calori GM, Tagliabue L, Mazza E et al. Tibial pilon fractures: which method of treatment? Injury 2010; 41: 1183–1190.
15. ABC of Emergency Radiology. Chan O (ed.) 3rd edn. Wiley Blackwell, 2013.
16. Weinberg AM, Jablonski M, Castellani C et al. Transitional fractures of the distal tibia. Injury 2005; 36: 1371–1378.
17. Anwar R, Nicholl JE. Non union of a fractured os trigonum. Injury Extra 2005; 36: 267–270.

Regularly overlooked injuries

- Lisfranc subluxations.

- Fatigue fractures involving the 2nd or 3rd metatarsals.

- Avulsion fracture of the base of the 5th metatarsal—overlooked on ankle radiographs.

The standard radiographs

Protocols vary. In the UK a two view series is commonplace: **AP and Oblique.** Elsewhere, and in the USA, a three view series is common practice[1,2]: **AP, Oblique**, and a **Lateral**.

Abbreviations

AP, anterior-posterior; MT, metatarsal.

Normal anatomy

The bones of the midfoot form an arch. As a consequence several of the tarsal bones, specifically the three cuneiform bones and the bases of the metatarsals, overlap on both the AP and oblique projections. The individual bones can be separated from one another when the AP and oblique radiographs are examined as a complementary pair.

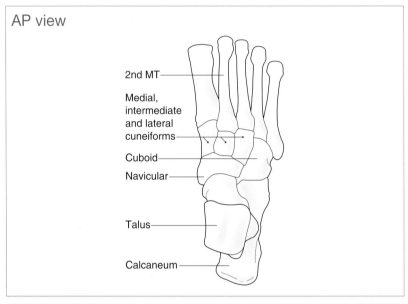

AP view

- 2nd MT
- Medial, intermediate and lateral cuneiforms
- Cuboid
- Navicular
- Talus
- Calcaneum

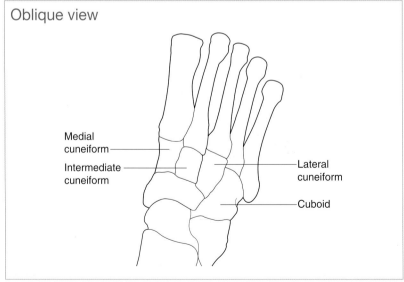

Oblique view

- Medial cuneiform
- Intermediate cuneiform
- Lateral cuneiform
- Cuboid

The cuneiform mortice and the Lisfranc joints

The base of the 2nd metatarsal is held in a mortice created by the three cuneiform bones. This mortice helps to prevent lateral slip of the bases of the metatarsals during weight bearing.

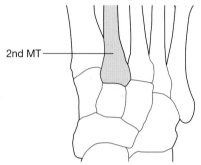

Alignment of 2nd metatarsal and the intermediate cuneiform. May appear "notched".

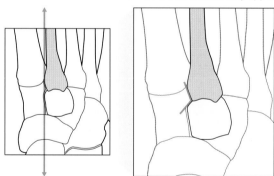

Alignment of 3rd metatarsal and the lateral cuneiform. May appear "notched".

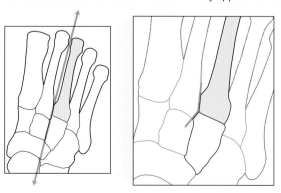

Analysis: the checklists

Analysis of the images will be influenced by the clinical findings such as the precise site of swelling, bruising, tenderness and pain.

The AP radiograph

Check :

1. Metatarsal and phalangeal shafts.

2. The Lisfranc joints. Always ask yourself... does the medial margin of the base of the 2nd metatarsal align with the medial margin of the cuneiform bone?

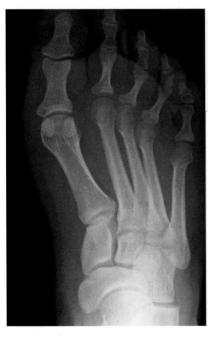
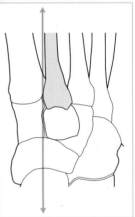

AP view.

Metatarsal shafts—normal. 2nd metatarsal aligns correctly with the intermediate cuneiform bone.

The oblique radiograph

Check:

1. Metatarsal shafts.

2. The Lisfranc joints. Does the medial margin of the base of the 3rd metatarsal align with the adjacent cuneiform bone?

3. The hindfoot bones and the hindfoot–midfoot articulations.

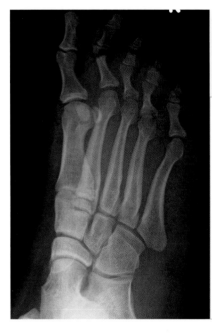

Oblique view.

Metatarsal shafts—normal.
3rd metatarsal aligns
correctly with the lateral
cuneiform bone.

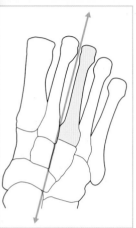

The lateral radiograph

Check:

1. Base of the 5th metatarsal.

2. The hindfoot bones and the midfoot articulations.

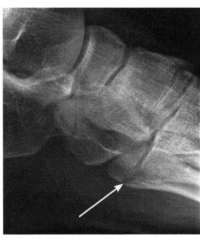

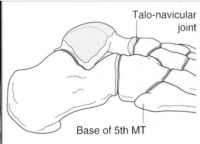

Lateral view.

Base of 5th metatarsal—fracture (arrow).

Midfoot articulations—normal.

The common fractures

Metatarsals and phalanges

- Very common. Some 35% of all foot fractures are metatarsal injuries[3]. In general, detection of a fracture involving any of the medial four metatarsals is easy.

- As many as 70% of all metatarsal fractures involve the 5th metatarsal[2].

Base of the 5th metatarsal

A fracture of the tuberosity represents an avulsion injury resulting from contraction of the peroneus brevis muscle and the pull of the plantar aponeurosis. It is caused by a plantar flexion–inversion injury.

A patient presenting with a twisted ankle: careful clinical examination of the base of this metatarsal will indicate when radiography of the foot, not the ankle, is necessary.

Potential pitfall: The normal unfused apophysis at the base of the 5th metatarsal is present in all children. It should not be misinterpreted as a fracture.

Helpful rules:

An avulsion fracture is situated either transverse or oblique to the long axis of the 5th metatarsal.

The normal childhood apophysis lies away from the articular surface and its long axis is aligned in a direction which is almost parallel with that of the shaft of the metatarsal.

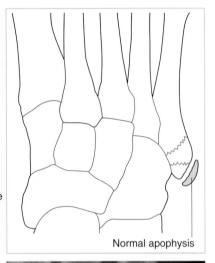

Normal apophysis

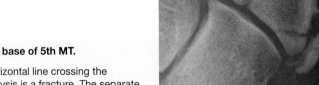

Injured base of 5th MT.

The horizontal line crossing the metaphysis is a fracture. The separate pieces of bone represent a normally developing apophysis.

Fatigue (march/stress) fractures

These injuries are frequently missed, misdiagnosed, mistreated, and misunderstood[4].

The 2nd and 3rd metatarsals are most commonly affected.

Radiographs are only abnormal when the fracture is well established. Abnormalities may not be visible for two or more weeks after the onset of symptoms.

If clinical suspicion of a fatigue fracture is high and the initial radiographs appear normal, it is worth considering a radionuclide bone study. Localised increase in uptake of the radiopharmaceutical in the context of a relevant history is diagnostic of a fatigue fracture. Alternatively, in (say) an elite athlete or footballer a similar suspicion would justify an MRI which would quickly confirm or exclude a fatigue fracture.

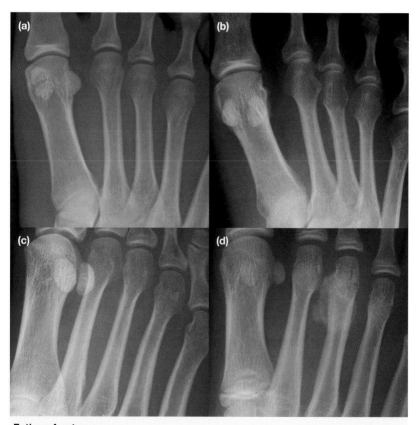

Fatigue fractures.

Four radiographic patterns may be present: (a) Normal; (b) Transverse or oblique crack (3rd metatarsal); (c) Faint periosteal reaction or fluffy callus (3rd metatarsal); and (d) Profuse callus (3rd metatarsal).

Infrequent but important fractures

Tarsal bone fractures

Midfoot tarsal bone fractures are uncommon, frequently resulting from high energy trauma. A major injury will be clinically obvious.

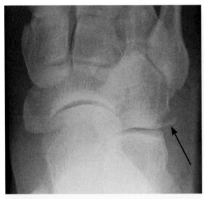
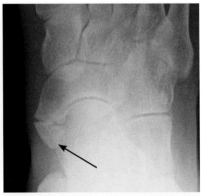

A fragment is detached from the lateral aspect of the cuboid (arrow). All the other bones and joints are normal.

Not a fracture. This is a very common normal finding (arrow). It is an accessory ossicle (os naviculare).

Base of the second, 3rd, or 4th metatarsal

Any fracture, whether a major fracture or a very small flake, at any of these sites will signal that there might be a major injury to a tarsometatarsal joint (a Lisfranc joint). See pp. 302–303.

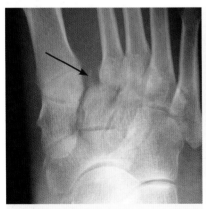
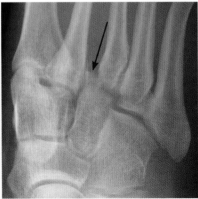

A fragment (arrow) has been detached from the base of the 2nd metatarsal. The base of this metatarsal has subluxed laterally.

A large fragment (arrow) is detached from the base of the 3rd metatarsal. The shaft of the 3rd metatarsal (ie the distal fragment) has subluxed laterally.

Jones fracture[1,2,4–6]

Two different fractures involve the proximal shaft of the 5th metatarsal: the very common avulsion injury (p. 298), and the much rarer but clinically important Jones fracture. It is important not to confuse these two fractures.

Jones fractures do not result from a simple avulsion injury.

The Jones fracture was first described by an orthopaedic surgeon, Robert Jones. He sustained the injury and subsequently published his experience[7]. Descriptions of this fracture in the literature are often confusing.

Clarification: a Jones fracture is a transverse fracture that lies distal to the styloid process of the fifth metatarsal, ie distal to the articulation between the bases of the 4th and 5th metatarsals. Characteristically it is positioned within 1.5 cm of the tuberosity.

A Jones fracture occurs as an acute injury, or, alternatively, following repeated stress affecting this metatarsal. Consequently some Jones fractures are fatigue fractures.

- The acute version results from a vertical or mediolateral force acting on the base of the metatarsal.

- The fatigue fracture version results from chronic overloading on the metatarsal, commonly in young athletes.

Delayed union or non-union are common problems, especially with a Jones fatigue fracture. In an elite athlete fixation with an intramedullary screw is often required.

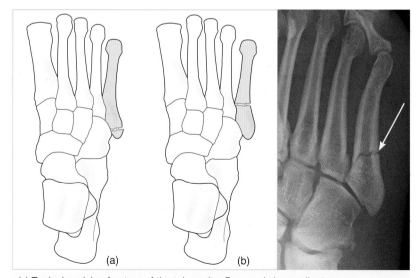

(a) Typical avulsion fracture of the tuberosity. Prognosis is excellent.

(b) Jones fracture (arrow). Non-union is a relatively common complication.

Dislocations/subluxations

Direct trauma commonly results in metatarsophalangeal or interphalangeal joint dislocations. These do not cause any difficulty in terms of diagnosis.

Injury to the tarsometatarsal joints[5,8–11]

Infrequent but very important. Walking and weight-bearing depend on the accurate alignment of the tarsometatarsal joints (see p. 295). Even a very slight subluxation requires meticulous reduction/management in order to preserve or restore function.

- Traumatic subluxations at the bases of the metatarsals (ie Lisfranc injuries) will be overlooked unless the normal alignment of the bones is carefully assessed. The radiographic appearance is often subtle. Always ask two questions:

  1. On the AP view does the medial margin of the base of the 2nd metatarsal align with the medial margin of the intermediate cuneiform?

  2. On the oblique view does the medial margin of the 3rd metatarsal align with the medial margin of the lateral cuneiform?

- Subluxation at a Lisfranc joint can occur with or without a fracture.

- Suspect a tarsometatarsal subluxation whenever a fragment of bone—however small—is detached from the base of any of the medial four metatarsals.

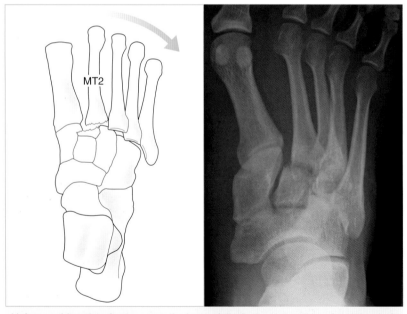

Lisfranc subluxation: fracture near the base of the 2nd metatarsal has freed the shaft of this bone from the restraining cuneiform mortice. Lateral slippage of the metatarsal bases has occurred in this patient.

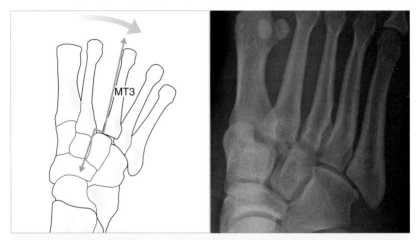

Lisfranc subluxation: the ligaments holding the 3rd metatarsal to the lateral cuneiform bone have been ruptured. Consequently, the 3rd metatarsal has subluxed laterally. The answer to question (2) at the botton of p. 296 is "No".

The reasons why some Lisfranc subluxations are overlooked on the radiographs[8–10]:

- Medical: failure to inspect the radiographs carefully.

- Medical: ignoring the importance of a tiny flake of bone avulsed from the base of the 2nd or 3rd metatarsal. A tiny flake is a big warning.

- Technical: the subluxation may have temporarily reduced because the radiograph is taken with the patient supine and not weight bearing. Apply this rule: whenever there is clinical concern regarding a possible Lisfranc injury and the radiographs appear normal then repeat the radiographs whilst weight bearing. Alternatively, CT or MRI imaging will be diagnostic[11].

Terminology[8,9]:

J. Lisfranc was a surgeon in Napoleon's army. He devised a forefoot amputation that took less than one minute to perform on soldiers who had frostbite or other injury. The amputation was through the tarsometatarsal joints. His imagination and skill has been rewarded by this series of eponyms.

- *Lisfranc joint or joints*: the tarsometatarsal joints

- *Lisfranc joint complex*: a description used by some when referring to the tarsometatarsal articulations.

- *Lisfranc injury*: a low-impact midfoot sprain. It is relatively common in athletes including American football players.

- *Lisfranc subluxation*: a high energy injury resulting in subluxation at a Lisfranc joint.

Pitfalls

Sesamoids and accessory ossicles

Numerous small bones are present on foot radiographs, and can be erroneously read as fracture fragments.

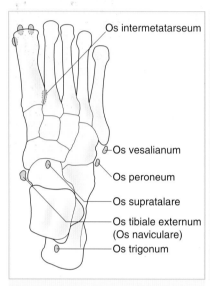

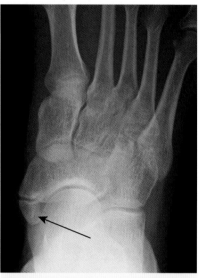

The most common sesamoid bones and the os naviculare.

The os naviculare (arrow). Also known as the os tibiale externum.

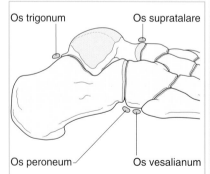

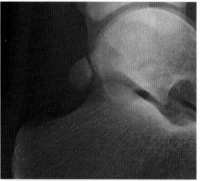

Three sesamoid bones and the os trigonum. These are the normal bones that cause concern or are questioned most frequently.

Another common accessory ossicle is the os trigonum. It lies posterior to the talus. Sometimes the ossicle is fused to the talus.

Apophysis

Normal apophysis at the base of the 5th metatarsal read as avulsion fracture (p. 298).

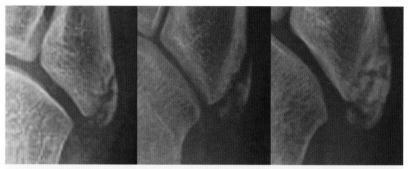

Normal apophyses. 100% of children have this apophysis. It usually ossifies as a single entity, but it may show multicentric ossification as in these three examples.

Epiphyseal clefts[12,13]

Defects or clefts occur normally in some epiphyses. They close around puberty. The basal epiphysis of the proximal phalanx of the great toe is a relatively common site. These clefts must not be confused with fracture lines.

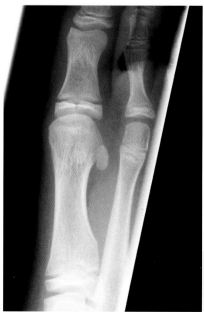

A cleft epiphysis.

A normal anatomical variant. This is the most common site of a cleft epiphysis.

An unrelated abnormality can cause distraction

Careful history taking and clinical examination is crucial to the correct assessment of the radiographs. Sometimes an unrelated abnormality will distract the unwary.

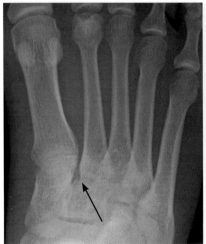

Injured midfoot.

The irregular and fragmented head of the 2nd metatarsal is not a recent injury. In this particular patient it could distract the unwary. It is a Freiberg's infraction. The important injury is at the base of the 2nd metatarsal where there is subluxation (arrow) at the Lisfranc joint.

Freiberg's infraction: flattening and fragmentation of the head of the metatarsal. Often associated with swelling, tenderness and pain. Most commonly seen in young women. Its aetiology remains obscure.

An error/pitfall[8-10] that needs repeated emphasis…

A foot is injured and an injury to a Lisfranc joint is a clinical possibility but the joint appears normal on the radiographs. An injury to the ligaments could still be present if spontaneous reduction of a subluxation has occurred. Remember that the radiographs are obtained as non weight-bearing images and the joint is not under the stress that occurs when the patient is standing. Weight-bearing views (or CT or MRI) should be obtained when there is continuing clinical concern in relation to a Lisfranc joint.

References

1. Berquist TH. Imaging of the foot and ankle. 3rd ed. Lippincott Williams and Wilkins, 2010.
2. Zwitser EW, Breederveld RS. Fractures of the fifth metatarsal; diagnosis and treatment. Injury 2010; 41: 555–562.
3. Spector FC, Karlin JM, Scurran BL, Silvani SL. Lesser metatarsal fractures. Incidence, management and review. J Am Podiatry Assoc 1984; 74: 259–264.
4. Anderson EG. Fatigue fractures of the foot. Injury 1990; 21: 275–279.
5. Prokuski LJ, Saltzman CL. Challenging fractures of the foot and ankle. Radiol Clin North Am 1997; 35: 655–670.
6. Shereff MJ, Yang QM, Kummer FJ et al. Vascular anatomy of the fifth metatarsal. Foot Ankle 1991; 11: 350–353.
7. Jones R. Fracture of the base of the fifth metatarsal bone by indirect violence. Ann Surg 1902; 35: 697–700.
8. Hatem SF. Imaging of Lisfranc injury and midfoot sprain. Radiol Clin North Am 2008; 46: 1045–1060.
9. Punwar S, Madhav R. Subtle Lisfranc complex injury: when not to trust normal Xrays. Injury Extra 2007; 38: 250–254.
10. Sherief TI, Mucci B, Greiss M. Lisfranc injury: How frequently does it get missed? And how can we improve? Injury 2007; 38: 856–860.
11. Kalia V, Fishman EK, Carrino JA, Fayad LM. Epidemiology, imaging, and treatment of Lisfranc fracture-dislocations revistied. Skel Radiol 2012; 41: 129–136.
12. Keats TE, Anderson MW. Atlas of normal Roentgen variants that may simulate disease. 9th ed. Elsevier, 2012.
13. Harrison RB, Keats TE. Epiphyseal clefts. Skel Radiol 1980; 5: 23–27.

18 Chest

Normal anatomy

Analysis: the checklists

Ten clinical problems

The chest X-ray (CXR)

A comprehensive description of the information that can be provided by the CXR requires a textbook all of its own.

Our companion book ***The Chest X-Ray : A Survival Guide***[1] will assist you to get the very best from this, the commonest radiological investigation in an Emergency Department (ED).

In this chapter we focus on the ten most common clinical questions that are asked of a CXR in the ED.

The standard radiographs

PA CXR. A lateral CXR in selected cases.

Abbreviations

CTR, cardiothoracic ratio;
CXR, chest X-ray;
LLL, left lower lobe;
LUL, left upper lobe;
LVF, left ventricular failure;
ML, middle lobe;
PA, posterior-anterior;
RLL, right lower lobe;
RUL, right upper lobe;
T3, the 3rd thoracic vertebra.

Normal anatomy

Frontal CXR—the lungs

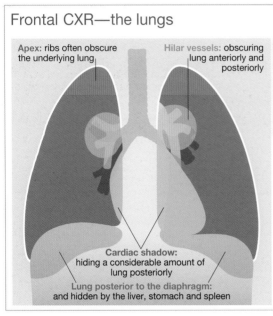

Apex: ribs often obscure the underlying lung

Hilar vessels: obscuring lung anteriorly and posteriorly

The tricky hidden areas.

The four areas where small (and large) lung lesions are overlooked.

Cardiac shadow: hiding a considerable amount of lung posteriorly

Lung posterior to the diaphragm: and hidden by the liver, stomach and spleen

Frontal CXR—lung markings

Normal lung markings are solely due to vessels and to nothing else. The normal bronchial walls, normal interstitium, and normal lymphatics are not visible.

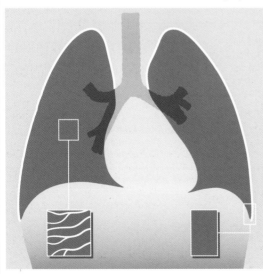

There is a complete absence of any lung markings in the lung immediately adjacent to each costophrenic angle.

In this peripheral part of the lung the normal vessels are simply too small to be visualised.

If this area shows detectable markings, then interstitial disease, or oedema, is likely[1].

Frontal CXR—hila

The hilum is the site at which the bronchi and vessels enter or leave the lung.

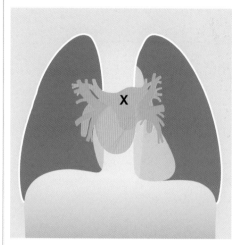

The two hila are approximately the same size and of very similar density.

The hilar shadows are due to pulmonary arteries and pulmonary veins. X marks the main pulmonary trunk.

Blue = pulmonary trunk and pulmonary arteries;
Red = pulmonary veins;
Lilac = part of left atrium.

Frontal CXR—cardiothoracic ratio

Most normal hearts have a cardiothoracic ratio (CTR) of less than 50% when assessed on a PA chest radiograph obtained in full inspiration[2].

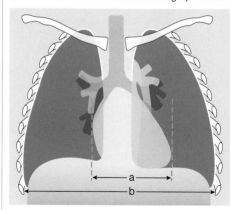

Measuring the CTR.

Two lines are drawn tangential to the outermost aspects of the right and left sides of the heart and the maximum cardiac width is measured.

The transverse diameter of the thorax is measured as the maximum internal width of the thoracic cage (ie inner cortex of rib to inner cortex of rib).

a/b < 50%.

Cardiac silhouette. The left and right borders of the heart are well defined by the surrounding air in the lungs.

Lateral CXR—the lobes of the lung

The two fissures in the right lung divide the lung into three lobes.

The single fissure in the left lung divides the lung into two lobes.

The oblique fissure on each side is propeller shaped and consequently we only, and very occasionally, see a part of a fissure on a normal lateral CXR.

On the other hand, we will see most of the horizontal fissure on the lateral CXR because it is straight. We will often see this fissure on the frontal CXR for the same reason.

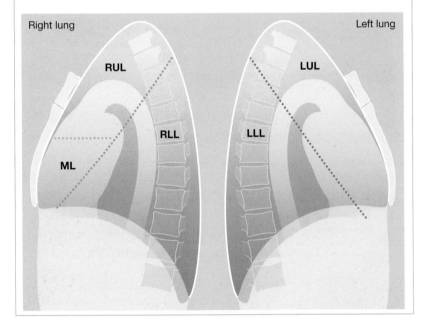

Lateral CXR—skeletal shadows

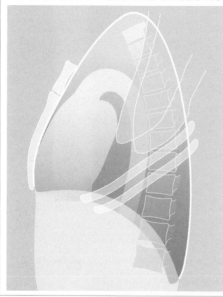

The scapula shadows (blue) are usually evident... but rarely create any difficulties.

The oblique shadows of the ribs are always evident.

The vertebrae are always seen.

Lateral CXR—three normal appearances

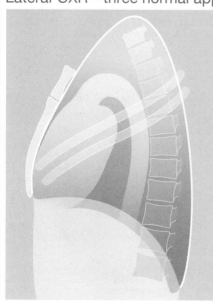

A normal lateral CXR will show three normal features relating to the two lungs (which project one over the other):

(1) The vertebral bodies gradually appear blacker as you look from T3 down to T12...
"grey at top; black at bottom".

(2) Both domes of the diaphragm are clearly visualised. Note that the anterior aspect of one dome (the left dome) fades away because the heart is positioned on this part of the dome.

(3) There is no abrupt change in density over the cardiac shadow. (Of course, any overlying rib shadows need to be discounted).

311

Analysis: the checklists

The frontal CXR

Four steps underpin accurate analysis.

1. Check whether the CXR is a PA or an AP radiograph and whether it was obtained erect or supine. An AP CXR will magnify the heart shadow; a supine CXR will alter the position of pleural air or pleural fluid.

2. Check whether there is an adequate inspiration. A small inspiration alters the normal appearance of the heart and lung bases.

3. Direct your initial analysis to your primary clinical concern.
    Is your primary concern: a left sided pneumothorax? A right sided pleural effusion? A coin lodged in the oesophagus?

4. Now you can assess the radiograph in an organised and systematic manner. As follows:

    ❏ Is the heart enlarged?

    In an adult, the cardiothoracic ratio (CTR) should be < 50% on a PA CXR (see p. 309).

    ❏ Are both domes of the diaphragm clearly seen and well defined?

    If part of a dome is obscured, suspect pathology in the adjacent lower lobe.

    ❏ Are both heart borders clearly seen and well defined?

    If not, there is a high probability of pathology in the immediately adjacent lung.

    ❏ Are the hila normal... position, size, density?

    ❏ Check the tricky hidden areas of the lung: both apices, behind the heart shadow, around each hilum, below the diaphragm (see p. 308).

    ❏ Are the bones normal?

    ❏ Finally, ask yourself once again:

    Have I addressed this patient's particular clinical problem?

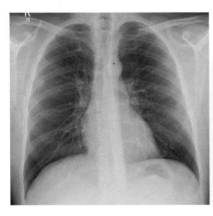

Normal PA CXR.

▪ Good inspiration.

▪ Heart size normal.

▪ Both domes of the diaphragm well defined.

▪ Both heart borders well defined.

▪ Hila unremarkable.

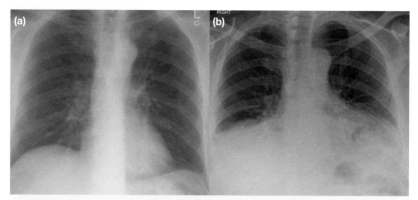

Is there an adequate inspiration? PA CXRs of the same patient: (a) is a good inspiration; (b) is a very poor inspiration. In (b) the heart appears enlarged and the lung bases hazy with crowding of vessels. These appearances are bogus; they are due to the extremely poor inspiration. CXR (a) is normal.

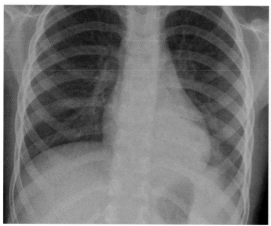

Are both domes of the diaphragm clearly seen and well defined?

Both domes of the diaphragm will be well defined if the adjacent lung is normal. In this patient, presenting with chest pain and fever, much of the left dome is obscured. This is due to pus in the adjacent alveoli.

Diagnosis: left lower lobe pneumonia.

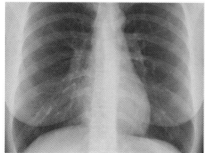

Are both heart borders clearly seen and well defined?

Both heart borders will be well defined if the adjacent lung is normal. In this patient with a cough and fever the right heart border is obscured because the air in the adjacent lung has been replaced by pus.

Diagnosis: middle lobe pneumonia.

The lateral CXR

Four questions underpin accurate analysis:

1. Are the vertebral bodies becoming blacker from above downwards?

   If not (ie they are becoming whiter or greyer) then suspect disease in a lower lobe or in a pleural space.

2. Are the domes of the diaphragm clearly visualised? Remember that one dome, the left dome, disappears anteriorly because the heart is tight up against it. If any other part of either dome is obscured—suspect consolidation or collapse in the adjacent lung.

3. Is there any abrupt change in density across the heart shadow?

   "An abrupt change in density" is likely to be a lung abnormality.

4. Have I correlated my findings on the lateral CXR with the frontal CXR appearances?

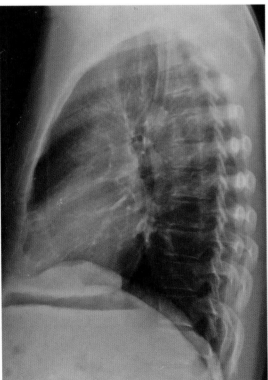

Normal lateral CXR.

- Vertebral bodies are "blacker" at the T9–T12 levels. Remember the rule: "grey at top; black at bottom".

- Both domes of the diaphragm are sharply defined.

- No abrupt change in density over the cardiac shadow.

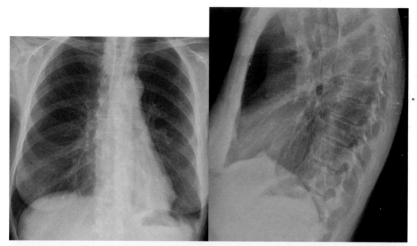

Female patient with cough and fever of recent onset. The lateral CXR is abnormal:
(1) The vertebral bodies appear whiter at the T9–T12 level; (2) only one dome of the
diaphragm is sharply defined. Conclusion: lower lobe pneumonia. The frontal CXR
confirms that the pneumonia is situated behind the heart in the left lower lobe.

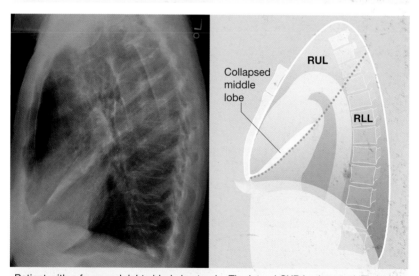

Patient with a fever and right sided chest pain. The lateral CXR is abnormal. The main
finding is that there is an *"abrupt change in density over the cardiac shadow"*. This
density is white, extends inferiorly from the hilum, and has sharp margins superiorly
and inferiorly. The density represents collapse within the middle lobe of the right lung.
This is shown in the explanatory drawing. (The dotted line indicates the position of
the oblique fissure in the right lung.)

Ten clinical problems

The full breadth of the radiology of thoracic disease as revealed by the plain CXR is addressed in our companion book *The CXR: A Survival Guide*[1]. We cannot cover that detail in this single chapter.

Instead, we will consider the ten clinical problems that account for well over 90% of all CXR requests made in the Emergency Department. We will take each problem in turn and pose a clinical question of the frontal CXR.

Question 1: Is there pneumonia (consolidation)?

Physical examination is not always sufficiently accurate on its own to confirm or exclude the diagnosis of pneumonia[3]. Many pneumonias will be obvious on the frontal CXR. Some are much more difficult to detect—the hidden pneumonias.

Detecting a hidden pneumonia

▨ Search for any evidence of a silhouette sign[1,2,4] on the CXR.

▨ Assess the mediastinal and diaphragmatic boundaries/borders.

▨ When a border is ill-defined, the precise site of a concealed area of consolidation is revealed. Sometimes the loss of a border is much more obvious than the actual air space density that occurs with a pneumonia.

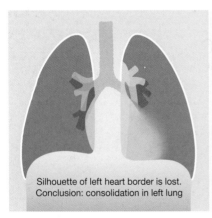

Silhouette of left heart border is lost.
Conclusion: consolidation in left lung

The silhouette sign. An intrathoracic lesion or density touching a border of the heart, aorta, or diaphragm will obliterate part of the border on the CXR[1,2].

Explanation: the borders of the heart and both domes of the diaphragm are visible on a normal CXR because the air in the lung contrasts with the water density of the heart and diaphragm. If lung air is replaced by pus (pneumonia) the immediately adjacent border will disappear or be ill-defined. This obliteration is termed the silhouette sign.

What does the word "consolidation" mean?

When lung alveoli fill with fluid (pus, water, or blood) there will be a shadow on the radiograph. Although the word "consolidation" is often used synonymously to imply that the shadow is an area of pneumonia, this is not strictly correct. There are other causes for air space shadowing (ie consolidation) and these include: pulmonary haemorrhage, pulmonary oedema, and fluid aspiration.

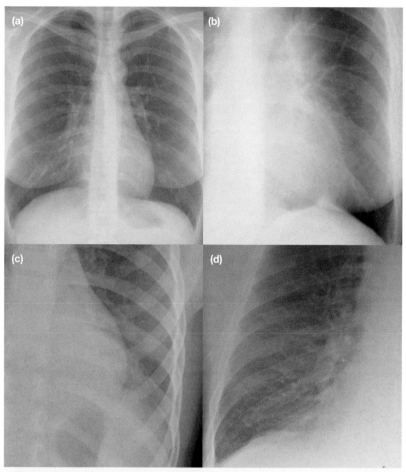

Hidden pneumonia: checking the borders

Partly ill-defined or absent	Suspect consolidation and/or collapse of the...
Right heart border	Middle lobe (a)
Left heart border	Left upper lobe (b)
Left dome of diaphragm	Left lower lobe (c)
Right dome of diaphragm	Right lower lobe (d)

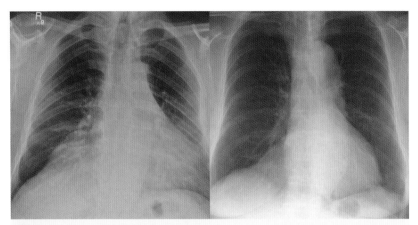

Silhouette sign—Pitfall. Mediastinal fat[1].

Some middle aged people accumulate a large collection of fat adjacent to the heart causing the heart border to be ill defined. The fat is of lower density than the water density of lung consolidation and this difference will help you to avoid this pitfall.
The patient on the left has lost the sharp silhouette of both the right heart border and of the right dome of the diaphragm. The patient on the right has lost the silhouette of part of the right dome of the diaphragm. In both cases the cause is a large collection of fat.

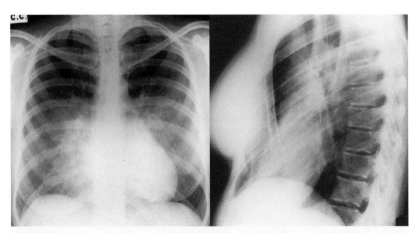

Silhouette sign—Pitfall. Depressed sternum.

The right heart border is effaced, and there is added density suggesting middle lobe consolidation. The lateral CXR shows the depressed sternum which is the cause of the grossly abnormal appearance on the frontal CXR[1]. The lungs are clear.

Question 2: Is there a pneumothorax?

An erect CXR obtained in full expiration is recommended. The normal lungs are more opaque (or slightly whiter) on an expiration CXR. Consequently, when a pneumothorax is present the air (black) in the pleural space contrasts with the adjacent (whiter) lung. This accentuation of the difference in contrast, as compared with an inspiration film, sometimes makes it slightly easier to detect a pneumothorax.

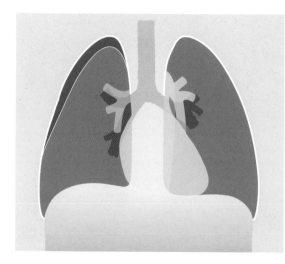

A pneumothorax shows three features on the erect CXR:

- A clearly defined line (ie the visceral pleura). This line parallels the chest wall.

- The upper part of this line will be curved at the lung apex.

- An absence of lung markings (ie vessels) between the lung edge and chest wall.

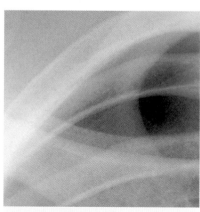

Shallow pneumothorax.
The visceral pleural line is visible.

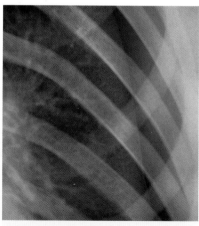

Pneumothorax. Note the well-defined line that represents the lung edge (ie the visceral pleura). Also, there are no vessels lateral to this line.

Supine CXR. In a severely injured patient the CXR will inevitably be obtained with the patient supine. On a supine CXR the pleural air will rise to the highest point in the pleural space—ie to the anterior aspect of the thorax. Consequently the lung base and the area around the heart need careful evaluation[4].

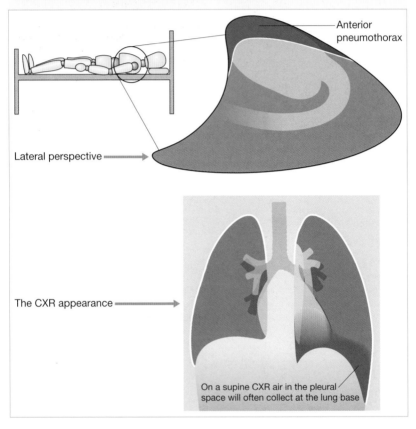

Anterior pneumothorax

Lateral perspective

The CXR appearance

On a supine CXR air in the pleural space will often collect at the lung base

Pitfall. An error rate of over 70% in detecting a pneumothorax by the trauma team when reading supine CXRs in the acute setting has been reported[5]. An upright CXR or, when this is not possible, either sonography or an early CT will be necessary when a pneumothorax is not evident but needs definite exclusion.

Pitfall. A skin crease in an infant or in the aged, overlying clothing, sheets, or intravenous lines can mimic a visceral pleural margin. The CXR should always be repeated after a rearrangement of the possible artefacts whenever there is any doubt as to the precise nature of a presumed lung edge.

Question 3: Are there signs of left ventricular failure (LVF)?

Look for cardiac enlargement and for lung and pleural changes.

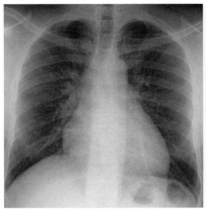

Cardiac enlargement.

Almost all patients with LVF have an enlarged heart. The occasional exception is a patient with an acute myocardial infarction.

Most enlarged hearts have a cardiothoracic ratio (CTR) over 50% when assessed on a PA CXR (p. 309).

The CTR is well over 50% in this patient.

Caveats:

- A CTR should not be read as abnormal:

    - on an AP CXR—because of magnification.

    - if the sternum is depressed, or if there is an exceptionally narrow AP diameter of the thorax.

    - in some elderly patients when the internal thoracic diameter is reduced because of bone (rib) softening.

- A heart may be enlarged despite a normal CTR. If the transverse cardiac diameter was very, very, narrow when the heart was normal, the enlargement that has occurred since then may not have reached 50% of the transverse diameter of the thorax.

- A few normal people (approximately 2%) have a CTR over 50%[2].

LVF; heart, lung and pleural changes. Erect PA, CXR

Early	Enlarged heart
	Oedema: poorly defined (slightly blurred) margins of the hilar vessels
	Oedema: septal lines (Kerley B lines)
	Small pleural effusions, usually bilateral
Later	Interstitial shadowing, and/or alveolar shadowing (florid oedema), and/or larger pleural effusions, usually bilateral.

Early LVF. Septal lines (Kerley B lines) caused by fluid in the interstitium. These short, straight lines reach the pleural surface and have this characteristic appearance at the lung base.

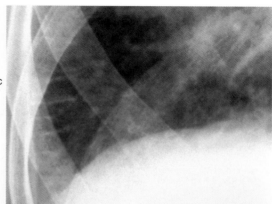

Early LVF. Small pleural effusions. Slight blunting of the costophrenic angles. Effusions in LVF are usually bilateral.

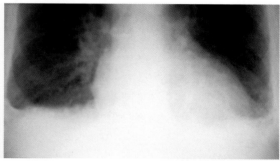

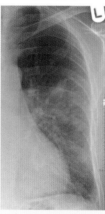

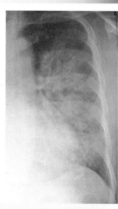

Interstitial oedema. The fluid lies mainly in the interstitium of the lung (ie oedema within the alveoli is less evident). Consequently, the shadowing is predominantly nodular and linear.

Extensive alveolar oedema. The fluid lies mainly within the alveolar air spaces (ie oedema lying in the interstitium is much less evident). Consequently the shadowing has a fluffy or cotton wool-like appearance.

322

Question 4: Severe asthmatic attack
—is there a complication?

The complications to look for are lung consolidation, lobar collapse, pneumothorax and pneumomediastinum.

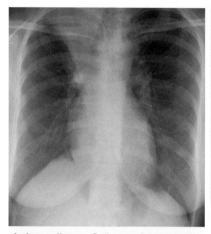

Lobar collapse. Collapse of the right upper lobe.

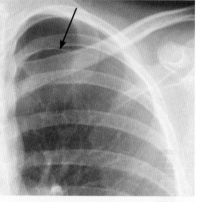

Pneumothorax. Air can dissect through the lung and in the region of the hilum it may enter the pleural space. The arrow indicates the visceral pleural line.

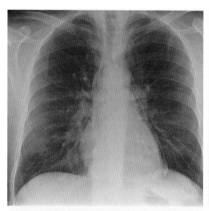

Pneumomediastinum. Streaks of air in the mediastinal soft tissues. The streaks may extend up into the neck. In this patient the air has dissected into the soft tissues around the left cardiac margin.

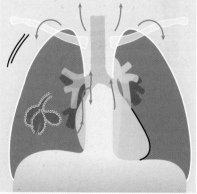

Pneumomediastinum explained. Air has dissected through the lung to the hilum and up into the neck. It can appear in the soft tissues of the chest wall. In addition, the dissecting air may outline a margin of the heart.

Question 5: Is there a pleural effusion?

Fluid in the pleural space can adopt several different appearances.

On the erect frontal CXR[1]

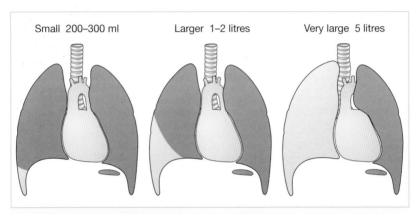

Small 200–300 ml   Larger 1–2 litres   Very large 5 litres

The commonest appearance is a meniscus at a costophrenic angle. It requires 200–300 ml of pleural fluid to efface the normal sharp sulcus between the diaphragm and the ribs. If the effusion is large, the entire hemithorax is opaque and the heart is pushed towards the normal side.

Other patterns also occur:

Top: Puddling in a subpulmonary position is relatively common. A **subpulmonary effusion** is usually easier to detect on the left side, where the puddle in the pleural space can cause the gastric air bubble to appear widely separate from the (apparent) superior margin of the diaphragm.

Bottom left: A linear (lamellar) effusion.

Bottom right: Fluid loculated in the pleural space. In this example— within the horizontal fissure.

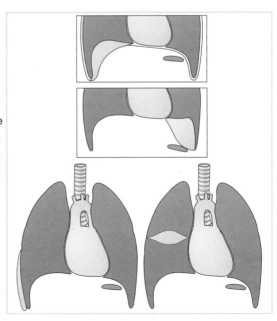

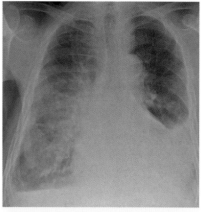

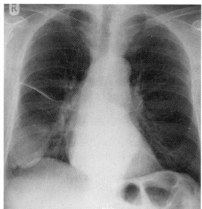

Small effusion on the patient's right side (a meniscus is evident).

A larger effusion is present on the left side... again, a meniscus appearance is evident. Note that the lung shadows are consistent with alveolar and interstitial oedema.

Encysted pleural fluid.

(1) In the horizontal fissure.
(2) Posteriorly in the pleural space. The latter has produced a "blob like" appearance (without a sharp superior margin) overlying the lower zone of the right lung.

On the supine CXR[1]

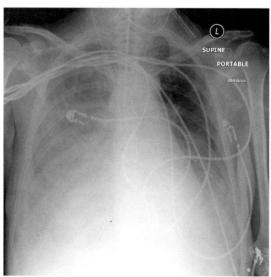

Pleural fluid on a supine CXR[1].

The fluid spreads to the most dependent site (ie to the posterior aspect of the pleural space). This causes the right hemithorax to appear greyer/whiter than the opposite side.

In this patient almost all of the shadowing over the right hemithorax is due to a large pleural effusion.

Question 6:
(a) Is there an aortic dissection?
(b) Is there a traumatic rupture of the aorta?

When assessing the mediastinum there are no absolute measurements that indicate abnormal widening on a frontal CXR.

Aortic dissection[4,6,7]

▨ The CXR is often normal.

▨ In the appropriate clinical setting mediastinal widening, with or without a left pleural effusion, is highly suggestive.

▨ Always compare the present CXR with any previous CXR, if available. An alteration to the mediastinum may be obvious.

▨ Clinical suspicion of a dissection must take priority over a normal CXR, and additional imaging becomes mandatory in all cases.

Traumatic rupture[8–10]

▨ 30% of patients with an aortic rupture have a normal CXR on presentation. If the CXR is normal, the level of clinical concern will determine whether an additional definitive radiographic examination (for example CT) is needed.

▨ A widened mediastinum does not necessarily indicate aortic rupture following blunt trauma to the chest. Tearing of small mediastinal veins is the most common cause of mediastinal widening on the CXR.

Pitfall.

In middle-aged and elderly patients, the aorta will often show age-related unfolding. Furthermore, on an AP projection an unfolded but otherwise normal aorta can be considerably magnified.

This patient has an unfolded aorta.

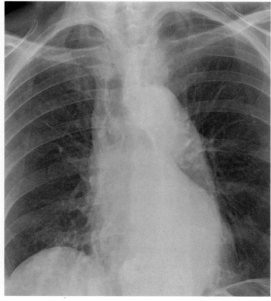

Question 7: Is there a rib fracture?

Oblique views of the ribs are not indicated following a relatively minor injury to the thorax. Clinical management is rarely altered by demonstration of a simple rib fracture. A frontal CXR is obtained solely to exclude an important complication such as a pneumothorax.

Pitfalls.

When recording a diagnosis of "no rib fracture", remember:

1. A fracture through a costal cartilage will not be visible on a CXR. Cartilage, unlike bone, is radiolucent.

2. A fracture through the bone may be present but it will not be detectable unless there is some displacement. Many rib fractures are initially undisplaced.

Question 8: Is there a cause for non-specific chest pain?

In many of these patients the pain remains unexplained and the CXR is normal.

Systematic analysis of the CXR (p. 312) will sometimes reveal an unexpected cause of the pain (eg pneumothorax, spontaneous pneumomediastinum[11], rib fracture).

The main pitfalls.

Over reading or under reading a CXR appearance.

- Example of over reading: an unfolded aorta read as an aortic dissection.

- Example of under reading: casual inspection overlooks an apical pneumothorax.

Question 9: Is there evidence of a pulmonary embolus?[1,4]

90% of emboli occur without pulmonary infarction and the CXR often appears normal.

Sometimes non-specific CXR findings are present, including: small areas of linear collapse; a small pleural effusion; slight elevation of a dome of the diaphragm.

Whenever a pulmonary embolus remains a clinical possibility then—whatever the CXR findings—the patient requires definitive imaging, usually a CT pulmonary angiogram.

Pitfall.

Unilateral lucency (ie hypertransradiancy) due to an area of reduced lung perfusion is well described with massive pulmonary infarction. It is a very rare finding. More commonly hypertransradiancy will have a technical cause such as patient rotation[1].

Question 10: Is there evidence of an inhaled foreign body?

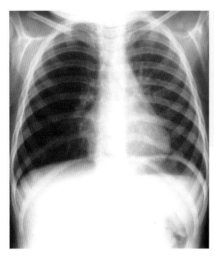

This patient had inhaled a peanut and attended the Emergency Department. This CXR is abnormal. It shows evidence of an obstructed bronchus. An additional CXR was obtained, following a particular manouvre, and that CXR provided confirmation of the obstruction. The peanut was removed.

The CXR analysis is provided on p. 30.

References

1. de Lacey G, Morley S, Berman L. The Chest X-Ray: A Survival Guide. Saunders Elsevier, 2008.
2. Goodman LR. Felson's Principles of Chest Roentgenology. 3rd ed. Saunders Elsevier, 2007.
3. Wipf JE, Lipsky BA, Hirschmann JV et al. Diagnosing pneumonia by physical examination: relevant or relic? Arch Intern Med 1999; 159: 1082–1087.
4. Hansell DM, Lynch DA, McAdams HP, Bankier AA. Imaging of Diseases of the Chest. 5th ed. Mosby Elsevier, 2010.
5. Ball CG, Ranson K, Dente CJ et al. Clinical predictors of occult pneumothoraces in severely injured blunt polytrauma patients: A prospective observational study. Injury 2009; 40: 44–47.
6. Jagannath AS, Sos TA, Lockhart SH et al. Aortic dissection: a statistical analysis of the usefulness of plain chest radiographic findings. Am J Roentgenol 1986; 147: 1123–1126.
7. Fisher ER, Stern EJ, Godwin JD et al. Acute aortic dissection: typical and atypical imaging features. Radiographics 1994; 14: 1263–1271.
8. Schnyder P, Wintermark M. Radiology of blunt trauma of the chest. Berlin. Springer-Verlag, 2000.
9. Mirvis SE, Templeton PA. Imaging in acute thoracic trauma. Semin Roentgenol 1992; 27: 184–210.
10. Gavelli G, Canini R, Bertaccini P et al. Traumatic injuries: imaging of thoracic injuries. Eur Radiol 2002; 12: 1273–1294.
11. Iyer VN, Joshi AY, Ryu JH. Spontaneous pneumomediastinum: analysis of 62 consecutive adult patients. Mayo Clin Proc 2009; 84: 417–421.

19 Abdominal pain & abdominal trauma

The AXR

Analysis: plain film checklists

The common problems

Infrequent but important problems

Appropriate imaging

- CT is frequently the optimum first line investigation.
- US is sometimes the optimum first line test.
- The AXR has a limited, occasionally useful, role.

Abbreviations

AXR, abdominal X-ray examination;
CT, computed tomography;
CT KUB, computer tomographic examination of the renal tract;
CXR, chest radiograph;
ED, Emergency Department, Emergency Room;
FAST, focussed abdominal sonography for trauma;
IVU, intravenous urogram;
US, diagnostic ultrasound/sonography.

The AXR—its usefulness

A patient with abdominal trauma does not require a plain abdominal radiograph (AXR). The AXR will not contribute to the clinical diagnosis and should be avoided.

The AXR is of limited value as a diagnostic tool in the evaluation of many patients presenting with an acute abdomen. This is largely because the abdominal contents are composed of soft tissue. Plain film radiography does not provide adequate soft tissue contrast discrimination to detect and differentiate between many of the numerous inflammatory and neoplastic intra-abdominal soft tissue pathologies. The AXR is not the right tool for the job. Consequently, it has been superseded by ultrasound and CT scanning which are highly accurate in terms of evaluating the various intra-abdominal soft tissues.

In present day clinical practice, the AXR is in the main limited to confirming a clinical suspicion of large or small bowel obstruction (as illustrated below), and demonstrating dangerous swallowed foreign bodies. Even so, CT will be selected as the first line imaging test in many cases of suspected intestinal obstruction, and also as the preferred and only imaging examination when renal colic is suspected.

What if the preferrred imaging investigations are not immediately available? Is there any point in requesting an AXR as a substitute imaging test? On the whole, no. You risk obtaining false reassurance from a seemingly normal AXR appearance. It is safer to rely on a detailed clinical history and a careful physical examination. Furthermore, an experienced pair of examining hands from a member of the surgical team will recognise the emergency case that needs to go to theatre.

The table on the right indicates the relatively few occasions when an AXR can be useful.

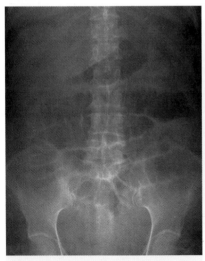

Distended small bowel. No large bowel gas. Diagnosis: small bowel obstruction.

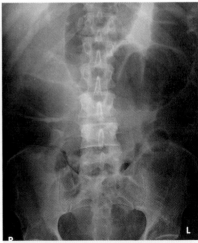

Gross distention of the large bowel extending as low as the sigmoid colon. Diagnosis: large bowel obstruction.

Radiology and abdominal pain

Clinical problem	The best tests	Is an AXR useful?
Small bowel obstruction	▨ CT—will often show the point of obstruction/cause	Yes. It will confirm the clinical impression in most cases.
Large bowel obstruction	▨ CT—will often show the point of obstruction/cause	Yes, to confirm the clinical impression.
Perforation	▨ Erect CXR ▨ CT	No
Appendicitis	▨ Clinical examination ▨ Ultrasound ▨ CT	No
Biliary Colic	▨ Utrasound	No
Cholecystitis	▨ Ultrasound	No. Will show calcified gallstones occasionally, but will not show wall thickening/inflammation.
Diverticulitis	▨ CT	No
Pancreatitis	▨ CT	No
Haematemesis	▨ Endoscopy	No
Acute lower gastrointestinal bleeding	▨ CT angiogram	No
Bowel ischaemia	▨ CT	No
Aortic aneurysm	▨ Clinical examination ▨ Ultrasound ▨ CT	No
Acute colitis	▨ Sigmoidoscopy	Yes. Will exclude toxic megacolon.
Constipation	▨ Clinical history & examination; rectal examination	No
Renal colic	▨ CT KUB	No. On its own it is imprecise and non-specific.

Analysis: plain film checklists

Erect CXR

In the context of a patient attending the Emergency Department with abdominal pain there are just two questions to ask of the CXR:

1. Does the erect CXR show any evidence of free air under the diaphragm?

2. Is there any evidence of pneumonia?

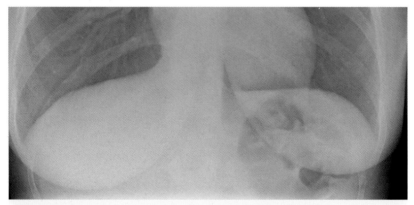

This erect CXR shows: normal lung bases and no free air under the diaphragm. The normal appearance of each lung is described on pp. 308–313.

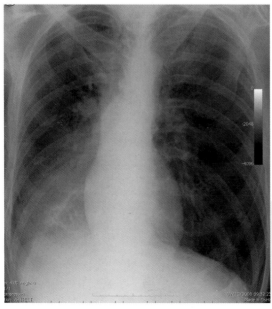

Abdominal pain. No specific diagnostic features from the history and clinical examination. The erect CXR reveals an extensive pneumonia in the right lower lobe.

Supine AXR

When analysing an AXR some normal features can be listed:

- Gas within the stomach may be seen as gas outlining the gastric folds in the left upper quadrant; there is rarely any gas seen in the small bowel.

- Normal gas patterns in the colon and rectum will vary. Sometimes segments of gas will be seen but no long continuous segments that are distended.

- No calcification overlying the liver or gall bladder, nor over the pancreas, kidney, ureters or urinary bladder.

- Calcification in the aorta may be age related and is common in the elderly; it will not show any localised bulge.

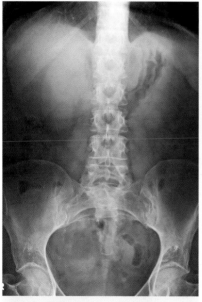

Supine AXR.

Normal features on this AXR: gastric folds/rugae outlined; faeces in the ascending colon; no bowel distension; no pathological calcification.

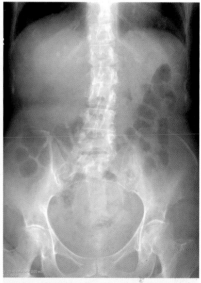

Supine AXR.

Elderly patient. Predominantly normal features on this AXR. Gas in an undistended large bowel (ascending, transverse, and descending colon); some age related calcification in the aorta. (The liver shadow might be prominent, but possible hepatomegaly is better assessed on palpation during the clinical examination.)

The common problems[1-10]

Both the likelihood of a particular diagnosis and the level of clinical concern will determine the specific radiological investigation that is selected. In some instances no imaging will be requested. The local availability of equipment or particular skills may also influence the choice of the first line test.

The following descriptions refer solely to plain film radiography; ie when a supine AXR or a CXR is obtained in the Emergency Department.

Non-specific abdominal pain

An erect CXR is primarily obtained in order to exclude a basal pneumonia or free air under the diaphragm. A supine AXR is not a useful test, because:

■ A normal AXR does not exclude serious pathology.

■ A good clinical history and physical examination are more useful than an AXR.

Following clinical examination the most useful imaging tests are CT or ultrasound. In the absence of these facilities, an AXR is unlikely to be better than the clinical examination performed by an experienced member of the surgical team.

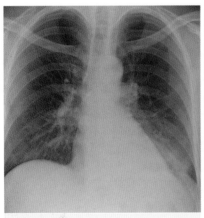

Erect CXR. Extensive pneumonia in the left lower lobe.

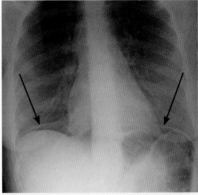

Erect CXR. Free air below both domes of the diaphragm (arrows). The lung bases are clear.

Pneumonia diagnosis

Pneumonia is a well recognised cause of acute abdominal pain, particularly in children. It might be unwise to place too great a reliance on the clinical examination of the chest alone as a means of excluding a pneumonia. A prospective survey[1] concluded:

"the traditional chest physical examination is not sufficiently accurate on its own to confirm or exclude the diagnosis of pneumonia".

334

Suspected perforation

The most useful radiograph is a well-penetrated erect CXR. An erect AXR is not indicated as the CXR is much more reliable in detecting free air. Very small quantities (as little as 1.0 ml) of free air can be demonstrated on an erect CXR[2].

If a patient is unable to sit up for an erect CXR then an alternative technique is employed: the patient reclines in the left-side-down decubitus position and a cross table AXR is obtained using a horizontal X-ray beam.

Other options:

- In some centres in North America, CT is requested as the first line investigation. CT is the most sensitive imaging test for diagnosing pneumoperitoneum. It is highly accurate, and it will often indicate the precise site of the perforation.

- In a few centres sonography is utilized for the detection of free intraperitoneal air[3]. Practitioners tend to follow a step by step protocol. As follows: plain radiography first; then ultrasound only in those in whom the plain radiograph (usually an erect CXR) is normal. CT is thus reserved for those occasions when ultrasonograhy still fails to make the diagnosis[6].

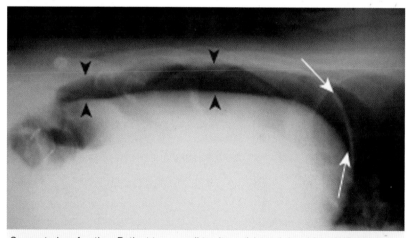

Suspected perforation. Patient too unwell to sit up. A lateral decubitus AXR with the patient lying on the left side. A large amount of free intraperitoneal air is shown (between the arrowheads) above the lateral surface of the liver. The air outlines the undersurface of the right dome of the diaphragm (arrows).

Suspected intestinal obstruction

The options:

1. CT.

   CT is highly accurate in demonstrating or excluding obstruction[4,5]. In addition, the precise site and probable cause of the obstruction can usually be defined. In an individual patient, the surgical team may well prefer CT as the first line imaging test, because of the excellent detail and additional information that will be provided.

2. Supine AXR.

   Some basic features will assist with diagnosis.

   ❏ *Dilated small bowel with an absence of colon gas* suggests a complete, or a nearly complete mechanical obstruction to the small bowel.

   ❏ *Dilated small bowel with gas in an undistended colon* suggests **either** an incomplete mechanical obstruction to the small bowel, **or** a localised adynamic (ie paralytic) ileus.

   ❏ *Dilated large bowel but no small bowel dilatation* suggests mechanical obstruction to the large bowel with a competent ileo-caecal valve.

   ❏ *Dilated large bowel with dilated small bowel* suggests **either** mechanical large bowel obstruction with an incompetent ileo-caecal valve, **or** a generalized adynamic (ie paralytic) ileus. The distinction is usually clinically obvious.

Pitfalls.

The supine AXR may appear normal—to the inexperienced observer—in two circumstances:

1. A very high small bowel obstruction.

2. Very occasionally the obstructed small bowel will distend with fluid and not with gas. Consequently there will not be the usual finding of multiple loops of bowel distended with gas.

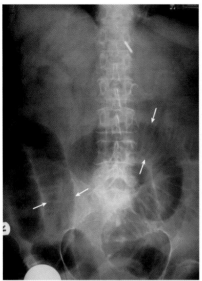

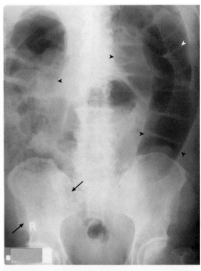

Colicky abdominal pain.

Dilated loops of small bowel (arrows). Some loops measure 50 mm in diameter (the upper limit of normal is 30 mm). Almost no gas within the large bowel. Mechanical small bowel obstruction.

Colicky abdominal pain.

Transverse colon and descending colon are dilated (arrowheads). A small amount of gas in the distal sigmoid. The caecum and ascending colon are also distended and contain faecal residue (arrows). These findings indicate a high grade mechanical obstruction in the distal descending colon or in the sigmoid colon. The absence of small bowel dilatation is due to a competent ileo-caecal valve. If the obstruction persists, then the small bowel will eventually become distended with gas.

Suspected constipation

The plain AXR is rarely of help in reaching a diagnosis of constipation as being the likely cause of abdominal pain. Because:

- The clinical history in relation to a change in stool frequency and consistency, together with a rectal examination, is usually diagnostic.

- The normal quantity of formed stool in the colon varies from person to person. A subjective quantification on the basis of the AXR appearances can be erroneous.

337

Suspected renal colic

The options:

1. Unenhanced multidetector CT, often referred to as a CT KUB.

    The CT KUB is now established as the preferred imaging test when renal colic is suspected[5–9]. It is an accurate and quick examination and there is no need for intravenous contrast medium injection.

2. Sonography.

    A case has been made that in female patients presenting with flank pain and suspected renal colic, sonography should be the initial examination in order to detect the presence of hydronephrosis[6]. This alternative approach is (a) based on consideration of the CT radiation dose to the ovaries and (b) because sonography is so good at detecting other pathologies deep in the female pelvis that may account for the patient's symptoms.

3. AXR plus sonography.

    Others have suggested that patients should have an AXR and ultrasound as a combination examination and if negative that CT should be reserved for the patient who does not subsequently improve on conservative management[10]. The addition of the AXR has been found to improve the accuracy of diagnosis of renal colic, ie when compared with ultrasound as the solitary examination[10].

4. Limited intravenous urography.

    Carried out as a two film examination: A plain AXR will be diagnostic when there is an obvious opaque calculus in the line of the renal tract. It is less helpful if the film (image) appears normal. A calculus might be obscured by superimposed bone, or confused with a pelvic phlebolith, or might simply be insufficiently radio-opaque to be seen. Although 90% of renal calculi contain calcium, less than 50% are visible on an AXR. Consequently, a single additional AXR at 10 minutes after the intravenous injection of contrast medium will be highly accurate in confirming or excluding the presence of a ureteric calculus. Normal excretion of the contrast medium together with undilated calyces and ureter will exclude the diagnosis of renal colic; delay in excretion on the painful side and/or calyceal/ureteric dilatation will confirm the diagnosis of renal colic.

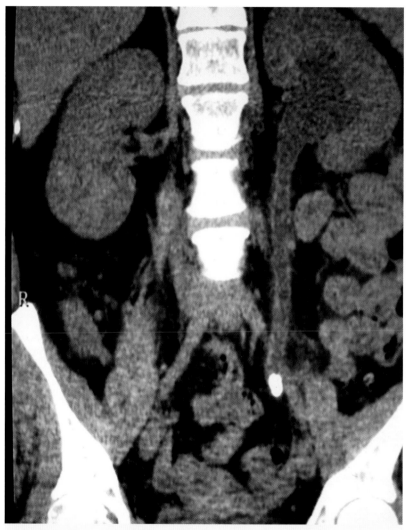

Clinical suspicion: acute left sided ureteric colic.

The patient was referred directly for a CT examination. The obstructing calculus in the lower third of the ureter is shown on this coronal reconstruction.

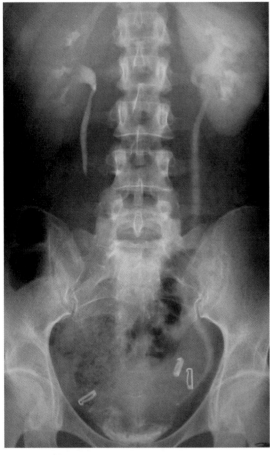

Clinical suspicion: acute left sided ureteric colic. Faint calcification in the true pelvis was seen on the supine AXR. This single radiograph obtained 10–20 minutes after the injection of contrast medium confirms that a calculus is causing ureteric obstruction.

Suspected acute biliary disease

Sonography is the first line imaging procedure whenever the suspicion is that of biliary colic or gall bladder disease.

Suspected abdominal aortic aneurysm/rupture

Sonography is the first line investigation.

Suspected foreign body ingestion

The important roles of the CXR, the AXR and hand held metal detector scanning are described in Chapter 21 (Swallowed Foreign Bodies).

Infrequent but important problems

Blunt trauma to the abdomen

In patients who have sustained abdominal or pelvic trauma the rapid assessment of the injury is critical. Delay increases mortality and morbidity[11].

■ Plain abdominal radiography is not indicated when investigating a blunt or penetrating injury. Obtaining an AXR is strongly discouraged—it delays the useful investigations.

■ Recommendations in relation to imaging[11]:

❏ Haemodynamically stable patient: the need is to demonstrate or exclude an intra-abdominal injury. CT is the examination of choice.

❏ Haemodynamically unstable patient: the need is to establish that the assumed bleeding is intra-abdominal. A FAST ultrasound examination is indicated. This test can be performed very quickly. If free fluid (blood) is detected then the patient can proceed to theatre for surgery.

Focussed abdominal sonography for trauma (FAST).

FAST is an abbreviated and protocol-designated form of ultrasound assessment that seeks only to demonstrate whether intraperitoneal or pericardial fluid is present or is increasing. It does not seek to define the exact site of injury. Carrying out a FAST study (after appropriate training) has been shown to be well within the capabilities of residents and registrars working in the Emergency Department[12–14].

Penetrating injury to the abdomen

■ *Haemodynamically stable patient*: If the surgeon does not elect to proceed immediately to surgery for wound exploration then CT is the most useful imaging test. CT will demonstrate organ damage.

■ *Haemodynamically unstable patient*: requires immediate surgery not imaging.

References

1. Wipf JE, Lipsky BA, Hirschmann JV et al. Diagnosing pneumonia by physical examination: relevant or relic? Arch Intern Med 1999; 159: 1082–1087.
2. Miller RE, Nelson SW. The Roentgenologic demonstration of tiny amounts of free intraperitoneal gas: experimental and clinical studies. Am J Roentgenol 1971; 112: 574–585.
3. Chen SC, Yen ZS, Wang HP et al. Ultrasonography is superior to plain radiography in the diagnosis of pneumoperitoneum. Br J Surg 2002; 89: 351–354.
4. Smith JE, Hall EJ. The use of plain abdominal X rays in the emergency department. Emerg Med J 2009; 26: 160–163.
5. Maglinte DDT, Kelvin FM, Rowe MG et al. Small bowel obstruction: optimizing radiologic investigation and non-surgical management. Radiology 2001; 218: 39–46.
6. Patatas K, Panditaratne N, Wah TM et al. Emergency Department imaging protocol for suspected acute renal colic: re-evaluating our service. Brit J Radiol 2012; 85: 1118–1122.
7. Kennish SJ, Bhatnagar P, Wah TM et al. Is the KUB radiograph redundant for investigating acute ureteric colic in the non-contrast enhanced computed tomography era? Clin Rad 2008; 63: 1131–1135.
8. The Royal College of Radiologists. iRefer: Making the best use of clinical radiology. London. The Royal College of Radiologists, 2012. [http://www.rcr.ac.uk/content.aspx?PageID=995]
9. British Association of Urological Surgeons (BAUS) guidelines for acute management of first presentation of renal/ureteric lithiasis. 2008. http://www.bauslibrary.co.uk/PDFS/BSEND/Stone_GuidelinesDec2008pdf
10. Ripolles T, Agramunt M, Errando J et al. Suspected ureteral colic: plain film and sonography Vs unenhanced helical CT. A prospective study in 66 patients. Eur Radiol 2004; 14: 129–136.
11. Jansen JO, Yule SR, Loudon MA. Investigation of blunt abdominal trauma. BMJ 2008; 336: 938–942.
12. Lingawi SS, Buckley AR. Focused abdominal US in patients with trauma. Radiology 2000; 217: 426–429.
13. Weishaupt D, Grozaj AM, Willmann JK et al. Traumatic injuries: imaging of abdominal and pelvic injuries. Eur Radiol 2002; 12: 1295–1311.
14. Ingeman JE, Plewa MC, Okasinski RE et al. Emergency physician use of ultrasonography in blunt abdominal trauma. Acad Emerg Med 1996; 3: 931–937.

20 Penetrating foreign bodies

The standard radiographs

Foreign body in soft tissue

■ Two radiographs—angulated so that bone does not obscure the injured site.

Orbital foreign bodies

■ Two frontal projections: upward and downward gaze.

Alternative imaging to consider

Soft tissue foreign bodies

■ Superficial: sonography.

■ Deeply penetrating: CT or MRI.

Orbital foreign bodies

■ CT or MRI.

Regularly overlooked foreign bodies

■ Glass hidden by bone.

■ Deeply penetrating FBs.

Abbreviations

CT, computer tomography;
FB, foreign body;
MRI, magnetic resonance imaging;
PA, posterior-anterior.

Appearances on plain radiographs

Glass

All glass is radio-opaque. Visibility of glass is not dependent on its lead content[1,2].

The radiographic density of the different types of glass does vary. Imaging technique is important. A soft tissue exposure is essential.

Zooming on a digital image is often necessary, otherwise very small fragments are easily overlooked.

Metal

Most metals are radio-opaque. A notable exception is aluminium.

Wood or plastic

Only occasionally will wood be visualised[3–5]. A splinter might be well defined on a radiograph if the fragment has paint on its surface.

Why is wood almost non-opaque on a radiograph?

■ **Explanation**: the detection of a foreign body is dependent on the atomic numbers of its constituent atoms in contrast to those of human soft tissue. Wood and soft tissue are both largely composed of carbon and other atoms with similar, low, atomic numbers. Therefore they are not readily differentiated by the X-ray beam.

In clinical practice it is best to assume that all splinters, thorns, and fragments of plastic will be non-opaque on a radiograph.

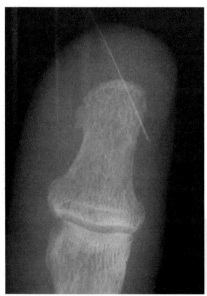

This splinter of wood was only visible because it had a thick coat of paint on its surface. It is usually very difficult to visualise wooden splinters or thorns on a radiograph.

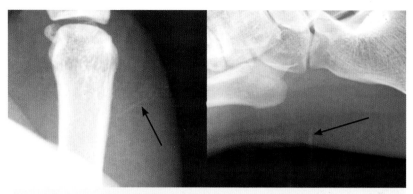

Wood splinters are often invisible, or barely visible, on a radiograph.
On the left, a wood splinter (arrow); on the right, a toothpick (arrow).

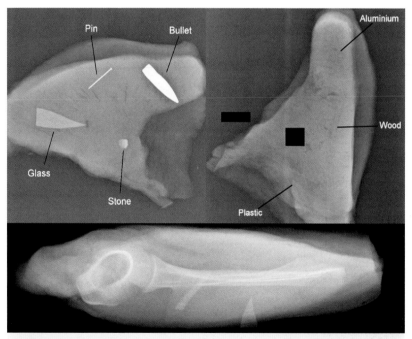

Visibility of penetrating foreign bodies. The top left image shows four different foreign bodies covered by soft tissue (turkey meat). The glass shard is from a broken picture frame. The top right image shows three other foreign bodies covered by turkey meat. All are invisible. The bottom image shows two pieces of glass buried in the soft tissues of a shoulder of lamb. Note that bone overlies part of one piece of glass and it is that portion of the fragment that is most difficult to visualise.

Suspected foreign bodies
Soft tissue laceration[6–8]

Foreign body detection

First choice in the Emergency Department: plain radiography.

- Glass and metals (except for aluminium) well visualised.
- Wood, plastic and aluminium not visualised.

Back up options in specific cases:

- Sonography (ultrasound).
  - Glass, metal, wood and plastic well visualised.
  - But… operator dependent, and will detect superficial foreign bodies only.
- CT.
  - Most foreign bodies are well visualised.
  - Wood can be difficult to visualise.
- MRI.
  - Wood shows up well.
  - A risky investigation if a foreign body is ferromagnetic.

Imaging pitfalls: Glass and metallic foreign bodies[2,3,8,9]

- **Pitfall (1):** Overlying bone on a radiograph will hide/obscure glass fragments including very dense shards. Project the site of injury away from bone. Two or more projections are required.

- **Pitfall (2):** If there has been high energy trauma, such as a fall from a height, a glass foreign body may be driven deep into the tissues and well away from the laceration. The precise history and circumstance in relation to the glass injury will determine if the radiographic field needs to be extended well beyond the laceration.

- **Pitfall (3):** With gun shot wounds the bullet (if there is no exit wound) can be situated far from the entry point. A wide radiographic field may need to be covered. On occasion, fluoroscopy can be helpful when searching for a missing bullet that has not been located on the original radiographs.

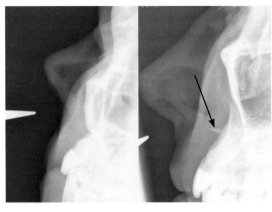

Glass wound to the face.

The left hand image shows the pointer indicating the site of the wound—but there is no evidence of a glass foreign body. The second image was taken with the maxilla rotated away from the site of injury, revealing a glass foreign body (arrow). Be careful: overlying bone will obscure or hide a glass foreign body.

Foreign body removal

Prior to surgical exploration it will sometimes be helpful if the precise position of a glass fragment or wooden splinter is shown beneath the skin. In these instances sonography can provide guidance at the time of removal. If a foreign body is situated deep in the soft tissues and sonography cannot provide the required information, then CT or MRI will often provide excellent localisation.

Orbital injury

Foreign body detection[10,11]

Most foreign bodies will be detected with slit lamp ophthalmoscopy.

Plain radiography, ultrasound, or CT will be of assistance in selected cases.

■ **Glass or metal fragments**

Plain film radiography is recommended.

■ **Wood or plastic fragments**

Sonography is recommended. The accuracy of detection is dependent on an experienced operator and the quality of the equipment. CT is an alternative to ultrasound and is the preferred investigation in some centres. CT is sensitive, shows the retrobulbar space better than ultrasound, and is less operator-dependent[10]. MRI is also available. It can be utilised when CT findings are uncertain[11]. A history of a ferromagnetic foreign body injury to the orbit is a contraindication to a MRI examination.

Penetrating foreign bodies

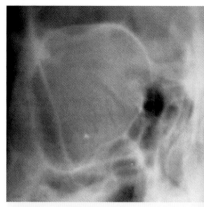

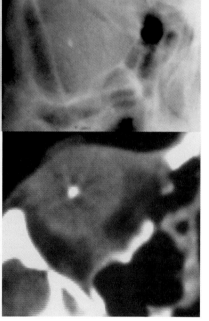

Orbital radiography.

Two frontal projections: downward gaze (top left) and then upward gaze (top right). Movement (or lack of movement) of a fragment on upward and downward gaze will indicate whether it is situated within or outside the globe.

CT is available should there be any lack of certainty as to the position of a foreign body after the plain films have been scrutinised. The CT image shown on the right is of a different patient.

Foreign body removal

Ultrasound or CT can provide accurate localisation prior to exploration of the orbit[10].

References

1. Tandberg D. Glass in the hand and foot. Will an X-ray film show it? JAMA 1982; 248: 1872–1874.
2. de Lacey G, Evans R, Sandin B. Penetrating injuries: how easy is it to see glass (and plastic) on radiographs? Br J Radiol 1985; 58: 27–30.
3. Hunter TB, Taljanovic MS. Foreign Bodies. Radiographics 2003; 23: 731–757.
4. Peterson JJ, Bancroft LW, Kransdorf MJ. Wooden Foreign Bodies. Am J Roentgenol 2002; 178: 557–562.
5. Horton LK, Jacobson JA, Powell A et al. Sonography and Radiography of soft tissue Foreign Bodies. Am J Roentgenol 2001; 176: 1155–1159.
6. Ginsburg MJ, Ellis GL, Flom LL. Detection of soft-tissue foreign bodies by plain radiography, xerography, computed tomography, and ultrasonography. Ann Emerg Med 1990; 19: 701–703.
7. Gilbert FJ, Campbell RS, Bayliss AP. The role of ultrasound in the detection of non-radiopaque foreign bodies. Clin Radiol 1990; 41: 109–112.
8. Wilson AJ. Gunshot injuries: what does a Radiologist need to know? Radiographics 1999; 19: 1358–1368.
9. Boyse TD, Fessell DP, Jacobson JA et al. US of soft tissue foreign bodies and associated complications with surgical correlation. Radiographics 2001; 21: 1251–1256.
10. Etherington RJ, Hourihan MD. Localisation of intraocular and intraorbital foreign bodies using computed tomography. Clin Radiol 1989; 40: 610–614.
11. Kubal WS. Imaging of orbital trauma. Radiographics 2008; 28: 1729–1739.

The most common foreign bodies

Infrequent but important foreign bodies

Dangerous injuries

- Coins may lodge in the oesophagus—slightly dangerous.
    - The CXR must include the neck.
- Button batteries may lodge in the oesophagus—highly dangerous.
    - The halo sign is important.
- Two magnets in the bowel—highly dangerous.
    - Use of a compass may be crucial.

Useful tools

- X-ray machine.
- Hand held metal detector.
- A compass.
- CT Scanner.

Abbreviations

AXR, abdominal radiograph;
BB, button battery;
CXR, chest radiograph;
ED, Emergency Department;
FB, foreign body;
HHMD, hand held metal detector.

The most common foreign bodies[1]

Children: coins

Radiography…

- An AP chest radiograph (CXR) to include all of the neck below the angle of the mandible.

- An abdominal radiograph (AXR) is not indicated[2,3].

Occasionally, a coin will lodge in the oesophagus. Some of these patients will be asymptomatic. An unrecognised coin can cause clinical problems including erosion of the mucosa which may result in an abscess or mediastinitis[4]. It is important to confirm that any swallowed coin has passed beyond the oesophagus. If the CXR is clear then the parents can be reassured that the coin will be passed within a few days.

Does the stool need to be checked? Sometimes a coin will be overlooked in the stool; the parents would be better advised to return to the Emergency Department (ED) only if the child becomes symptomatic.

Coin composition: coins in the UK and in the European Union are made of steel or alloys of various metals and sometimes coated with copper. In effect, these coins are inert. This does not apply worldwide. For example, in 1982 because of the cost of copper the one cent coin in the USA (commonly referred to as the penny) was minted with a mainly zinc core and a thin copper coating. Interaction between gastric acid and zinc can cause ulceration in the stomach. This possibility led to various scares and the consequent overuse of routine AXR. The penny constituents were not changed, but eventually a practical recommendation was made and widely adopted: if a USA penny has been swallowed and the CXR is clear then an AXR need only be obtained in a child who subsequently developes intestinal symptoms. The latter is an exceptionally rare occurrence.

Hand held metal detector (HHMD) scanning[5–7]

Consider this as an alternative to radiography. Advantages of a HHMD include:

- It eliminates the need for a CXR.

- There is no ionizing radiation.

- It is accurate and easy to use with minimal training.

- Patient and parent time spent in the ED is reduced.

- It is cost effective.

- Its efficacy is underpinned by a tried and tested diagnostic algorithm.

Pitfall. If using a HHMD, a definite history in relation to the swallowed foreign body being a coin is most important. If the history is uncertain and the foreign body could be a magnet or a cluster of magnets (see p. 359) then a false reassurance might be provided by the HHMD. A safety net: concern regarding a cluster of magnets masquerading as a swallowed coin can be eliminated by passing a compass over the abdomen[8]. The lack of compass movement will exclude a magnet.

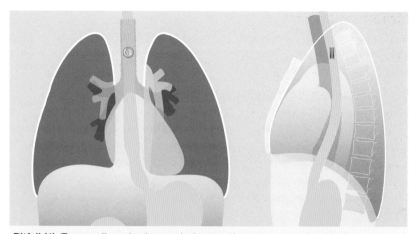

Pitfall (1). Two swallowed coins can lodge together at the same level in the oesophagus. The coins can overlap each other and appear as a single foreign body on the frontal CXR. A lateral CXR will demonstrate whether one or two coins are impacted.

Pitfall (2). The majority of retained coins are situated in the upper oesophagus[9–11] at the level of the cricopharyngeus muscle. An impacted coin can be missed if the whole neck below the level of the angle of the mandible is not included on the CXR.

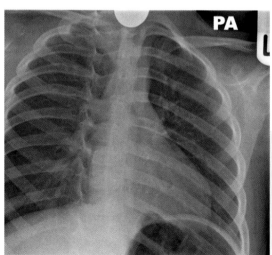

In this child the coin is only just included on the radiograph. The cardinal rule has not been followed…

"The CXR must include all of the neck below the angle of the mandible".

351

Swallowed foreign bodies

Adults: fish bones

Fish bones comprise more than 70% of all foreign body events that cause an attendance to some EDs[12,13]. Complications resulting from an impacted fish bone are rare but can be serious. These include: neck abscess, mediastinitis and lung abscess.

Fish bone impaction is very different to that of other impacted foreign bodies[14,15].

▦ Infrahyoid impaction is much less frequent. In one series[15] approximately 90% of fish bones were situated in the oro-pharynx, whereas approximately 90% of other foreign bodies (poultry bones, dentures, wood splinters, coins, pork bones and lamb bones) were impacted more distally in the laryngeal pharynx or upper oesophagus.

Radiography.

▦ The soft tissues of the oro-pharynx and down to the level of the hyoid bone are dense on the lateral radiograph. A lateral neck radiograph will rarely detect a fish bone impacted in these dense areas.

▦ The use of a lateral radiograph of the neck should be limited, selectively employed, and based on a diagnostic algorithm (see p. 353).

What to look for.

▦ The occasional fish bone that does impact below the hyoid bone.

▦ Evidence of a complication:

  ❏ Gas in the soft tissues, either as a streak or as a pocket, suggests perforation.

  ❏ Widening of the prevertebral soft tissues suggests an abscess.

Different fish bones have different radiographic densities[14,16,17]:

▦ **Readily visible**: cod, haddock, cole fish, lemon sole, gurnard.

▦ **More difficult to see**: grey mullet, plaice, monkfish, red snapper.

▦ **Not visible**: herring, kipper, salmon, mackerel, trout, pike.

Normal prevertebral soft tissue width:

▦ **Above C4 vertebra**: up to 7 mm.

▦ **Below C4 vertebra**: up to 22 mm.

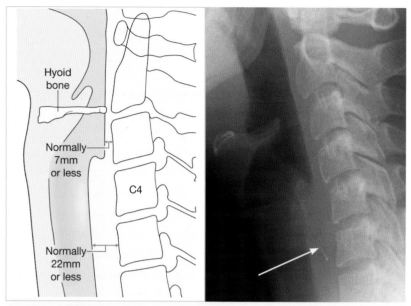

Fish bones. What to look for.

Check that the prevertebral soft tissue widths are within normal limits (left).

Look for a fish bone: faintly visible (arrow) anterior to the C6 vertebra (right).

A protocol for suspected fish bone impaction

1. Oro-pharynx examined with illumination.

    The vast majority of impacted fish bones will be visible. No radiography required.

2. If the fish bone is *not* seen in the oro-pharynx, then the next steps will depend on the level of clinical concern and on local guidelines. Possibilities:

    ❏ Request a lateral radiograph of the neck.

    Apply this rule: If the radiograph is normal and the patient is considered well enough to be sent home, then the patient should be told to re-attend the next day if symptoms are persisting. Patients who re-attend should be seen immediately by an ear, nose and throat specialist.

    ❏ Or… direct referral for endoscopy.

    ❏ Or… request CT of the neck.

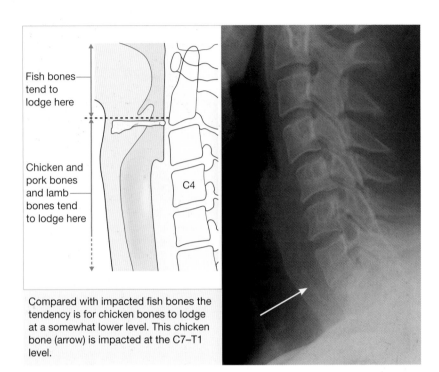

Fish bones tend to lodge here

Chicken and pork bones and lamb bones tend to lodge here

C4

Compared with impacted fish bones the tendency is for chicken bones to lodge at a somewhat lower level. This chicken bone (arrow) is impacted at the C7–T1 level.

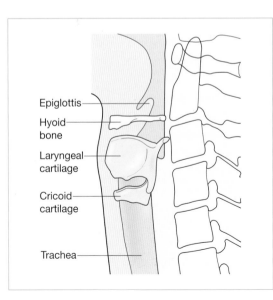

Epiglottis

Hyoid bone

Laryngeal cartilage

Cricoid cartilage

Trachea

Laryngeal and cricoid cartilages can ossify partly or almost entirely. There is no fixed pattern.

Partial ossification can lead to a false positive diagnosis of an impacted bone. Similarly an impacted bone may be dismissed as a partly ossified cartilage.

Careful analysis and linking that analysis to the clinical history is most important.

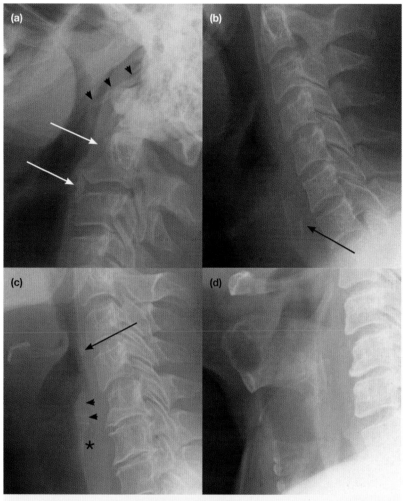

Beware. Normal calcifications and ossifications.

(a) Calcified stylo-hyoid ligament (arrowheads). Calcification (arrows) in relation to the anterior longitudinal ligament of the cervical spine.

(b) Calcification at the C6–C7 level (arrow) is ossification in the posterior aspect of the cricoid cartilage.

(c) Ossification in the triticeous cartilage (arrow); in the thyroid cartilage (arrowhead); in the cricoid cartilage (asterisk).

(d) Very extensive ossification/calcifications in the hyoid bone, the laryngeal cartilage, the cricoid cartilage, and in several tracheal rings.

Infrequent but important FBs

Sharp objects other than fish bones

Many sharp objects pass through the intestines without causing a problem. Nevertheless a sharp or pointed object may penetrate the oesophagus or the bowel. The presence of the swallowed object needs to be confirmed (or excluded).

Radiography:

- For metallic foreign bodies such as nails, needles, screws or razor blades a CXR and an AXR are indicated.

- For chicken, pork chop[18], or lamb bones a lateral view of the neck is indicated. Approximately 90% of these foreign bodies, when impacted, will be found to be lodged in the hypopharynx or upper oesophagus[15]. This is a very different position of impaction as compared with impacted fish bones (see pp. 352–353).

- Wood and plastic foreign bodies are radiolucent and will not be identified on a radiograph. If clinical suspicion is high (eg a swallowed and impacted pencil or toothpick) then CT, or a contrast medium swallow, or endoscopy, will be indicated.

- Aluminium (eg as in a drink can ring pull) is of very low radiodensity[19] and is rarely detectable on a radiograph. An aluminium ring pull (aka aluminium tab) will be detected by a HHMD[5-7]. Many countries have largely overcome the swallowed ring pull problem by producing ring pulls that remain attached to the can after the can is opened. Nevertheless, it is still possible to detach the ring pull from the can by wiggling it. Therefore the swallowing of ring pulls has not been eliminated entirely[20].

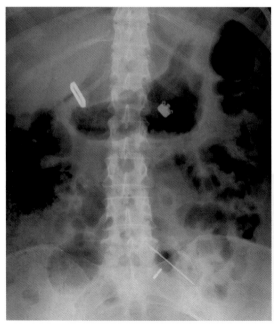

An AXR must be obtained whenever a sharp metallic object might have been swallowed.

A case of habitual foreign body ingestion. Four metallic foreign bodies are shown. The needle places the patient at risk of a perforation.

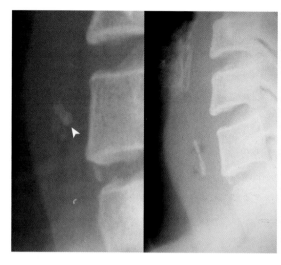

Be wary—the orientation of a foreign body can mislead.

Impacted chicken bone.

On presentation (far left) the bone (arrowhead) lay in a horizontal position and was not recognised.

Several days later (left) the bone lay vertically and is very easy to identify. Note the soft tissue swelling and faint bubbles of gas indicating an abscess around a perforation[1].

Why is a bowel perforation relatively infrequent?[10,21]

90% of swallowed foreign bodies pass through the intestine without any problem, and this includes many nails and razor blades.

Sharp metallic foreign bodies rarely perforate the bowel wall. The intestine resists perforation and laceration partly because it is lined with mucus, is very pliable, and when a sharp FB reaches the colon it becomes encased with faeces.

Travelling head first: a pin or needle will often pass through the intestine with the blunt end leading[21,22]. It has been suggested that ingested needles and pins tumble and turn until the blunt end faces forwards!

When perforations do occur they may be silent. A needle lying in the soft tissues outside of the bowel may be discovered years later on an AXR obtained for other reasons[21].

Swallowed foreign bodies

Button batteries[23–27]

An impacted button battery (BB) is a diagnostic and endoscopic emergency. If ingested, a CXR is crucial. Obtain it as soon as the patient arrives in the ED.

Most small size BB ingestions do not cause damage, provided the BB does not lodge in the oesophagus. The frequency of lodgement is increasing with widespread usage of the 20–25 mm diameter lithium batteries. A BB stuck in the oesophagus can cause serious mucosal injury. The damage is primarily caused by an electrical current that hydrolyzes soft tissue and results in liquefactive necrosis, not leakage of battery contents. Damage can occur very quickly, sometimes within one or two hours of lodgement[23,24]. Mucosal damage can result in oesophageal perforation, tracheoesophageal fistula, stricture formation, and death[24]. Rapid diagnosis and emergency removal of a lodged battery is essential.

Note: BBs can also cause a similarly serious injury if placed in the ear or nose[23,24,27].

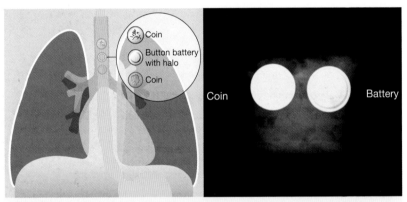

Those unfamiliar with the appearance of a BB on an AP CXR should look for the double rim or halo appearance of a BB as compared with the appearance of a small coin (ie no halo). This halo appearance is unique to a BB. The right hand image is a radiograph of a coin and a BB seen en face in ultrasound gel (soft tissue).

Pitfalls.

1. Unwitnessed ingestions in children are common and BB lodgement may initially cause non-specific symptoms. A high index of suspicion is necessary in those patients who are puzzlingly unwell and who may be prone to swallowing foreign bodies—ie little children.

2. If the CXR for a suspected foreign body does not include all of the neck below the angle of the mandible, a BB lodged high in the oesophagus can be missed.

3. A BB shown on a CXR can be misread as a coin or, occasionally, read as an external object such as an ECG electrode[23]. It is essential that those working in the ED always check whether or not any foreign body or metallic density overlying the oesophagus shows the incontrovertibly diagnostic halo sign.

Magnets[6,10–12,28]

Powerful rare earth magnets can be found in toys, jewellery items, beads, nose and tongue piercings, studs, desk toys, stress relievers, homeopathic and naturalistic aids, and other items such as bracelets used in folk medicine.

Swallowing magnets appears to be relatively common amongst autistic children with access to magnetic pieces[8].

The ED aim is to determine whether more than one magnet has been swallowed. If a child swallows more than one magnet and they pass through the pylorus then the separate pieces can attract each other across different bowel loops. Gut wall necrosis, perforation, fistulae, haemorrhage, and volvulus are potential and serious consequences. Alternatively, a child might swallow one magnet and another piece of metal to which it is attracted. This is also dangerous.

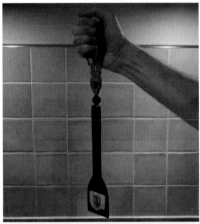

Small rare earth magnets are enormously powerful.

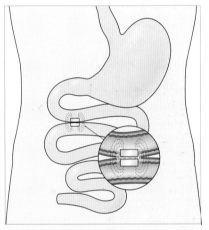

Two or more magnets in the bowel are highly dangerous.

Pitfalls.

1. On the AXR a cluster of magnets clumped tightly together across different bowel loops can be misread as a harmless necklace or other single object. Avoid this risk by putting a compass against the patient's abdomen[8]. If the compass indicates the object is a cluster of magnets, then it represents a surgical emergency.

2. Detection using a metal detector (p. 350) poses a similar risk. If there is uncertainty as to what has been swallowed, then a magnet detected by a HHMD might be assumed, erroneously, to be a coin. Placing a compass against the abdomen will assist. Lack of compass movement will exclude a magnet.

Swallowed foreign bodies

Large objects—dentures[29–31]

Radiographic appearance of dentures

▪ Methylmethacrylate is the acrylic plastic from which most dentures are constructed. It is radiolucent.

▪ Some, but not all, dentures will contain metal as a fixing or support and consequently will be radiographically visible when impacted[31].

▪ Note: Porcelain and plastic teeth are of very low radio-density[30].

A large object such as a dental plate or appliance may lodge in the cervical or thoracic oesophagus. If it remains impacted it may erode the mucosa and cause an abscess or mediastinitis. Radiography:

1. Well penetrated PA and lateral CXR, to include the neck.

2. If these images are normal, an AXR should be obtained.

3. If this image is normal, and the clinical history or symptoms remain suggestive, a barium swallow or endoscopy will be necessary.

A negative CXR does not exclude an impacted denture; not all dentures are radio-opaque.

Ingestion risk is not limited to partial dentures. Full (ie complete) dentures can be swallowed.

CT and MRI can help to identify acrylic dentures. However, image interpretation with these investigations is not always straightforward and can be very difficult[30].

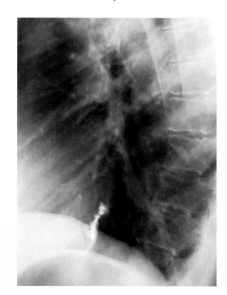

Denture impacted in the lower oesophagus. It was not identified on the frontal CXR. This lateral view was essential.

Hard plastic clips

Bread bag clip ingestion can cause intestinal perforation, stricture, or obstruction.

- Some countries have eliminated these bread bag clips and replaced them with tape; others have altered the design of the clip; others may still use these clips.

- The impaction mechanism is seemingly due to the prolapse of mucosa into the jaws of the clip. This impaction can erode the mucosa[32]. Complications from an impaction may be delayed and can occur years after the ingestion. Most cases of accidental ingestion of a bread bag clip occur in elderly and edentulous patients. The patient is usually unaware of having ingested this foreign body.

- Strong plastic bread bag clips are radiolucent and will not be detectable on a radiograph. The contribution from radiology is limited to providing assistance with the diagnosis of complications that may occur such as perforation or intestinal obstruction.

Bezoars[33]

A bezoar is ingested foreign material that accumulates within the gastrointestinal tract.

- The most frequent bezoars are phytobezoars (poorly digested fruit and vegetable fibres) and trichobezoars (ingested hair). Phytobezoars are the most common.

- Frequently there is a history of previous gastrointestinal surgery.

- Intestinal obstruction is a recognized complication.

Radiography:

- In general, plain film radiography is unhelpful (in diagnosing the likely cause) when a patient presents with bezoar induced intestinal obstruction.

- On the other hand, sonography or CT can assist with the rapid diagnosis of a bezoar as the cause of the intestinal obstruction[33].

References

1. Remedios D, Charlesworth C, de Lacey G. Imaging of foreign bodies. Imaging 1993; 5: 171–179.
2. Swallowed coins. Editorial. Lancet 1989; 2: 659–660.
3. Stringer MD, Capps SN. Rationalising the management of swallowed coins in children. Br Med J 1991; 302: 1321–1322.
4. Nahman B, Mueller CF. Asymptomatic oesophageal perforation by a coin in a child. Ann Emerg Med 1984; 13: 627–629.
5. Lee JB, Ahmad S, Gale CP. Detection of coins ingested by children using a hand held metal detector: a systematic review. Emerg Med J 2005; 22: 839–844.
6. Seikel K, Primm PA, Elizondo BJ, Remley KL. Hand-held metal detector localisation of ingested metallic foreign bodies; accurate in any hands? Arch Pediatr Adolesc Med 1999; 153: 853–857.
7. Ramlakhan SL, Burke DP, Gilchrist J. Things that go beep: experience with an ED guideline for use of a HHMD in the management of ingested non-hazardous metallic foreign bodies. Emerg Med J 2006; 23: 456–460.
8. CDC. Gastrointestinal injuries from magnet ingestion in children. United States, 2003–2006. MMWR 2006; 55: 1296–1300.
9. Koirala K, Rai S, Shah R. Foreign Body in the esophagus: comparison between adult and pediatric population. Nepal J of Med Sci 2012; 1: 42–44.
10. Hunter TB, Taljanovic MS. Foreign Bodies. Radiographics 2003; 23: 731–757.
11. Chung S, Forte V, Campisi P. A review of pediatric foreign body ingestion and management. Clin Pediat Emerg Med 2010; 11: 225–230.
12. Nandi P, Ong GB. Foreign body in the oesophagus: review of 2394 cases. Br J Surg 1978; 65: 5–9.
13. Lue AJ, Fang WD, Manolidis S. Use of plain radiography and computed tomography to identify fish bone foreign bodies. Otolaryngol Head Neck Surg 2000; 123: 435–438.
14. Ritchie T, Harvey M. The utility of plain radiography in assessment of upper aerodigestive tract fishbone impaction: an evaluation of 22 New Zealand fish species. NZ Med J 2010; 123: 32–37.
15. O'Flynn P, Simo R. Fish bones and other foreign bodies. Clin Otolaryngol Allied Sci 1993; 18: 231–233.
16. Ell SR, Sprigg A, Parker AJ. A multi-observer study examining the radiographic visibility of fishbone foreign bodies. J R Soc Med 1996; 89: 31–34.
17. Davies WR, Bate PJ. Relative radio-opacity of commonly consumed fish species in South East Queensland on lateral neck X-ray: an ovine model. Med J Aust 2009; 191: 677–680.
18. Liu J, Zhang X, Xie D et al. Acute mediastinitis associated with foreign body erosion from the hypopharynx and esophagus. Otolaryngol Head Neck Surg 2012; 146: 58–62.
19. Valente JH, Lemke T, Ridlen M et al. Aluminium foreign bodies: do they show up on X-Ray? Emerg Radiol 2005; 12: 30–33.
20. Donnelly LF. Beverage can stay-tabs: still a source for inadvertently ingested foreign bodies in children. Pediatr Radiol 2010; 40: 1485–1489.
21. Rahalkar MD, Pai B, Kukade G, Al Busaidi SS. Sewing needles as foreign bodies in the liver and pancreas. Clin Rad 2003; 58: 84–86.
22. Ward A, Ribchester J. Migration into the liver by ingested foreign bodies. Br J Clin Pract 1978; 32: 263.
23. Litovitz T, Whitaker N, Clark L et al. Emerging battery ingestion hazard: clinical implications. Pediatrics 2010; 125: 1168–1177.
24. Lee SL. Recognition of esophageal Disc battery on Roentgenogram. Arch Otolaryngol Head Neck Surg 2012; 138: 193–195.
25. Litovitz T, Whitaker N, Clark L. Preventing battery ingestions: an analysis of 8,648 cases. Pediatrics 2010; 125: 1178–1183.
26. Litovitz T, Schmitz BF. Ingestion of cylindrical and button batteries: an analysis of 2382 cases. Pediatrics 1992; 89: 747–757.
27. Premachandra DJ, McRae D. Severe tissue destruction in the ear caused by alkaline button batteries. Postgrad Med 1990; 66: 52–53.
28. Oestreich AE. Danger of multiple magnets beyond the stomach in children. J Nat Med Assoc 2006; 98: 277–279.
29. Hashmi S, Walter J, Smith W, Latis S. Swallowed partial dentures. J R Soc Med 2004; 97: 72–75.
30. Haidary A, Leider JS, Silbergleit R. Unsuspected swallowing of a partial denture. Am J Neuroradiol 2007; 28: 1734–1735.
31. Abu Kasim NH, Abdullah BI, Mahadevan I, Yunus N. The radio-opacity of dental prostheses (fixed and removeable) on plain radiographs—an experimental study. Annals Dent Univ Malaya 1998; 5: 35–39.
32. Morrissey SK, Thakkar SJ, Weaver ML, Farah K. Bread Bag Clip ingestion. Gastroenterol Hepatol (NY) 2008; 4: 499–500.
33. Ripolles T, Garcia-Aguayo J, Martinez MJ, Gil P. Gastrointestinal bezoars. Sonographic and CT characteristics. Am J Roentgenol 2001; 177: 65–69.

Assess the radiographs in this chapter to test your knowledge and diagnostic skills.

Each patient attended the ED/ER following trauma or complaining of pain.

See if you can identify the injury or problem revealed in each radiograph.

Beware. Some of the radiographs may be normal.

Answers are on p. 380.

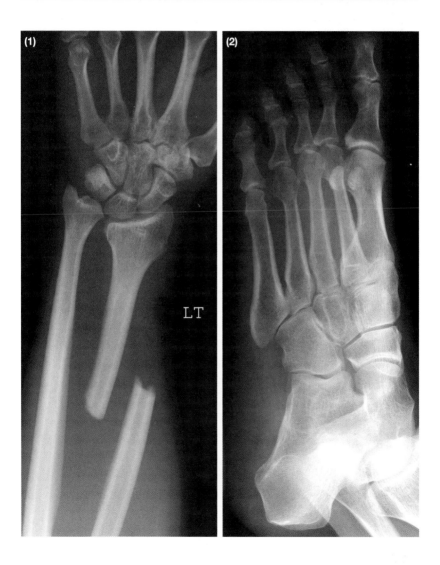

(1)

(2)

LT

(3)

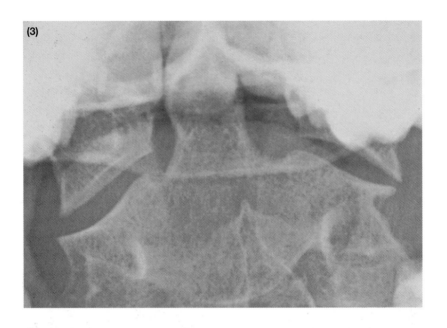

(4)

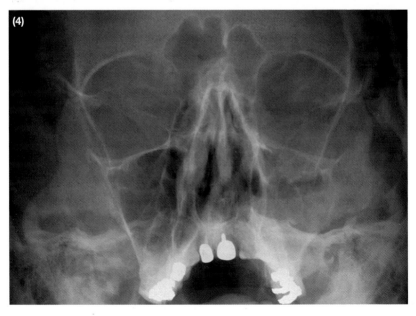

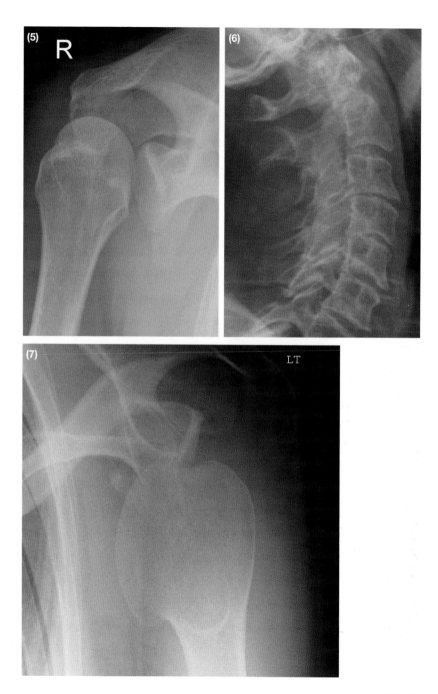

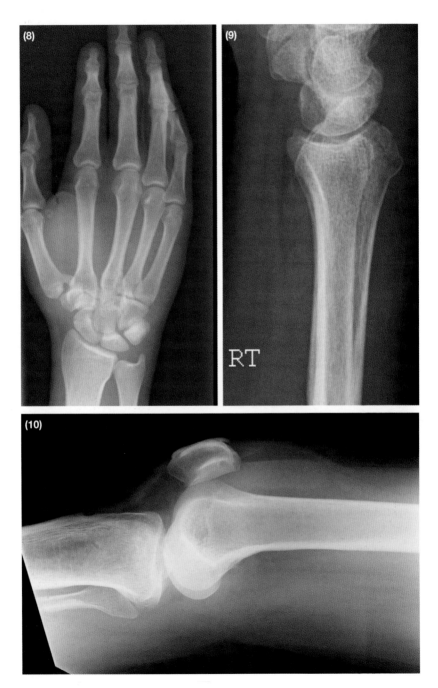

(8)

(9)

RT

(10)

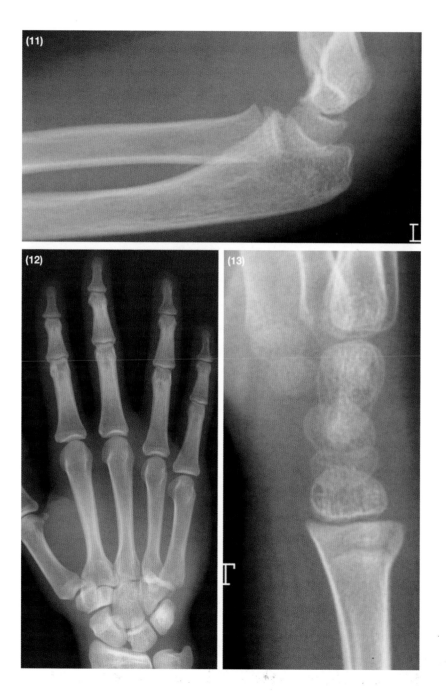

(11)

(12)

(13)

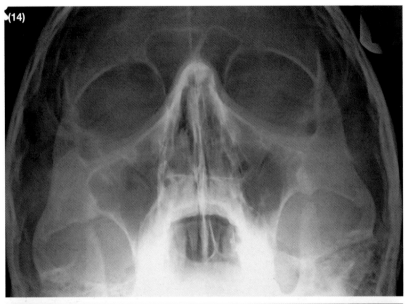

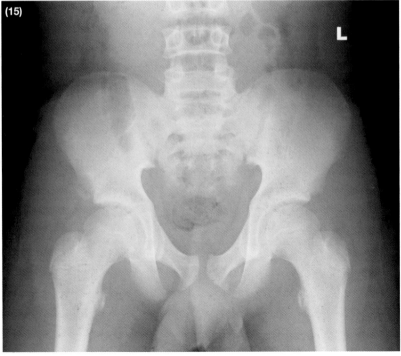

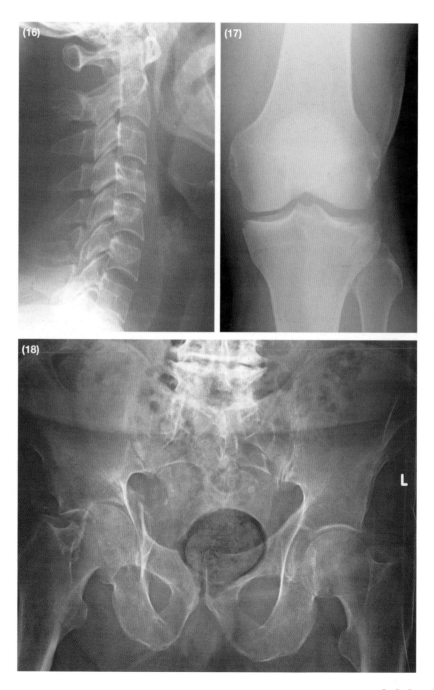

(16)

(17)

(18)

L

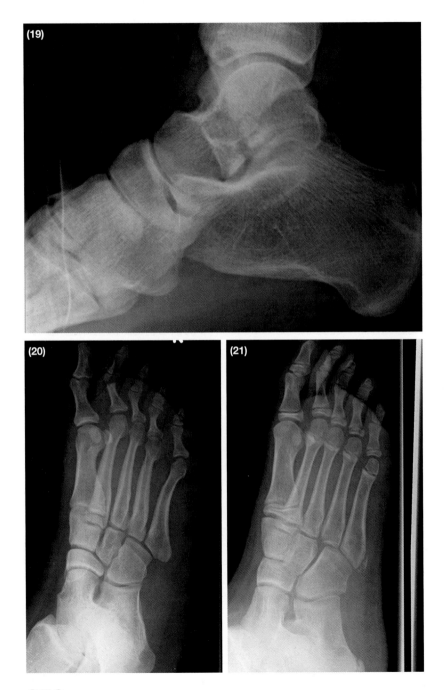

(19)

(20)

(21)

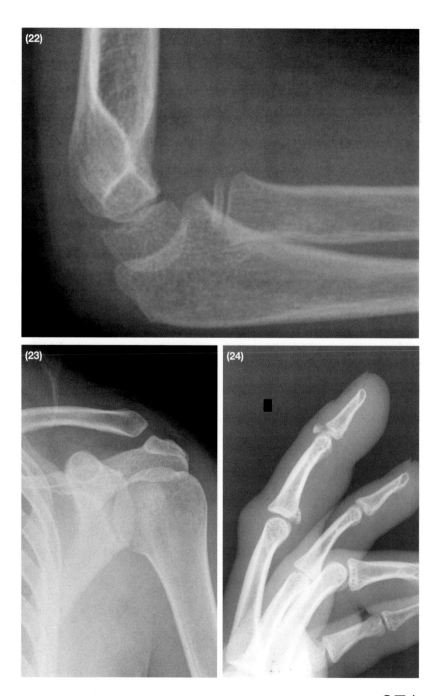

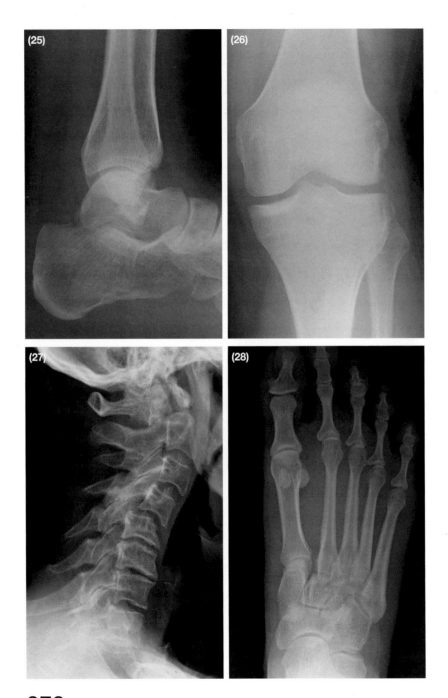

(25)

(26)

(27)

(28)

Glossary

Accident and Emergency Department. See: Emergency Department.

AP. Antero-posterior. Indicates direction of X-ray beam passing through the patient.

Axial radiograph aka axial projection or axial view. The X-ray beam is directed along a plane parallel to the long axis of the body. Example: axial view of calcaneum.

AXR (UK) aka KUB (USA). An abdominal radiograph.

Basal joint of the thumb. The 1st carpometacarpal joint (ie trapezium-metacarpal joint).

Baseball finger (USA). See: Mallet finger (UK)

Battered baby syndrome. See: Non-accidental injury (NAI).

Bayonet apposition. Describes the relationship of two fracture fragments when they lie next to, or adjacent to, each other rather than in end-to-end contact.

Bone bruise. Focal oedema and haemorrhage secondary to microfractures of the trabeculae. Can only be demonstrated by MRI. May take up to 4 months to heal.

Bowing fracture. See: Plastic bowing fracture.

Buddy strapping. See: Garter strapping.

Button battery aka **Disc battery**. Battery often used in watches and calculators.

Calcaneum aka Calcaneus.

Capitellum aka Capitulum.

Carpal navicular (USA) aka Scaphoid bone (UK)

Coffee bean shadow aka the reversed D shadow. A *Survival Guide* analogy/contrivance used to describe the anterior arch of the C1 vertebra as it appears on the lateral view of the cervical spine. This shadow is readily visible on all lateral radiographs and very approximately resembles a coffee bean. The analogy has been coined in order to assist the inexperienced doctor to identify and focus on this specific landmark shadow when analysing the anatomy at the C1/C2 articulation.

Compartment Syndrome. Fascial tissue surrounds and separates groups of muscles in the arms and legs. Within each fascial layer there is a confined space, termed a compartment. Swelling within a fascial compartment (ie oedema or blood) can compress the contained muscles, nerves, and blood vessels. Rising pressure can obstruct the blood flow to the compartment and cause permanent injury to the muscle and nerves. Consequently there can be extensive or complete replacement of the muscle by scar tissue.

CTR. Cardiothoracic ratio. A measurement. Indicates whether the heart is likely to be enlarged.

Decubitus position. Patient is reclining. Denotes that the patient is lying on his or her side. Implies that a horizontal beam radiograph has been obtained. A technique which can be used to demonstrate free intra-abdominal air or to confirm fluid in the pleural space.

Diaphysis. The shaft of a long bone. It merges with the metaphysis at either end. See: Epiphysis, Metaphysis, Physis.

Diastasis. Separation of normally adjacent bones with or without an associated fracture, or a separation at a site of fibro-cartilaginous union. Examples: the tibia and fibula at the ankle mortice; a sacroiliac joint; a skull suture.

Dorsal. Relating to the posterior (extensor) aspect of the body or of a body part (eg a limb). See: Ventral.

Emergency Department or ED (UK) aka Emergency Room or ER (USA), Accident Department (UK); Accident and Emergency Department (UK); Casualty (UK).

Glossary

Epiphyseal fusion aka Epiphyseal closure. The epiphysis when fully ossified merges with the metaphysis of the long bone. The age at which ossification and fusion occurs varies from bone to bone. There is a slight variation in the age at which fusions occur in males and females.

Epiphysis. The epiphysis forms the bone-end. It enlarges by growth of cartilage within the secondary centre adjacent to the growth plate. Gradually the epiphysis ossifies, and it eventually fuses to the metaphysis when the growth plate disappears. See: Epiphyseal fusion; Metaphysis.

Fluoroscopy (USA, UK) aka Screening (UK); Fluoroscopic screening. Viewing an area of anatomy on a screen or on a monitor utilising a machine which provides a real time X-ray image. Can (for example) be used to detect air trapping in a child who may have aspirated a foreign body. Also used to assist in the manipulation of fractures.

Garter strapping aka Buddy strapping. A method of immobilising some phalangeal fractures. The injured digit is strapped to an adjacent uninjured digit.

Growth plate aka Cartilaginous growth plate, Epiphyseal plate, Epiphyseal disc. The layer of cartilage between the metaphysis and epiphysis of an unfused long bone. Sometimes referred to as the Physis.

GSW. Gun shot wound.

Hip pointers. Contusions to the iliac crest causing pain, localized tenderness, and discomfort when weight bearing.

Horizontal beam radiograph aka Cross table radiograph. Denotes the orientation of the X-ray beam relative to the floor. The beam is parallel to the floor. This technique may be used to demonstrate a fluid level (eg in the suprapatellar bursa of the knee), or utilised when a patient should not be moved from the supine position (eg lateral cervical spine radiograph following trauma).

Insufficiency fracture. A fracture occurring as the result of a normal stress on an abnormal bone (eg a vertebral fracture occurring without trauma or a fall in an elderly patient who has osteoporosis). Aetiologically completely different from a stress fracture.

Intravenous urogram (IVU) aka Excretory urogram, Intravenous pyelogram (IVP).

Isotope investigation aka Nuclear medicine investigation, Radio-isotope study, Radionuclide scan, Scintiscan, Scintigraphy.

KUB (USA) aka AXR (UK). An abdominal radiograph.

Light of day appearance. The normal appearance of the 4th and 5th carpometacarpal joints on all posterior-anterior radiographs of the hand. It has a specific relevance to a patient who presents with a hand injury after punching a wall. Loss of the *light of day* appearance raises the strong probability of a dislocation of the affected carpometacarpal joint.

Lipohaemarthrosis. Liquid fat and blood within a joint demonstrable on a horizontal beam radiograph. Most commonly seen at the knee joint when marrow fat enters the joint via an intra-articular fracture and forms a fat-fluid level (FFL). Occasionally referred to as a fat-blood interface or FBI.

Lisfranc joints. The tarsometatarsal joints. Usually referred to in the context of a Lisfranc fracture dislocation; the most common dislocation or subluxation of the foot.

Lucent. Denotes a dark line, or dark area, on a radiograph. Commonly used as a descriptive term to indicate that a fracture is identifiable by a lucent line (or lucency).

Lytic. The opposite of sclerotic. Denotes an area on a bone radiograph which appears darker or blacker than the adjacent normal bone. The word lytic often implies bone destruction. Sometimes used as a synonym for lucent.

Mallet finger (UK) aka Baseball finger (USA). A flexion deformity of a distal interphalangeal joint with or without a fracture of the dorsum at the base of the terminal phalanx. The injury represents an avulsion of the extensor tendon.

March fracture aka Fatigue fracture, Stress fracture. It is common for the term March fracture to be used in reference (specifically) to a stress fracture of a metatarsal. A recognized complication during the training period for recruits into the army.

Metaphysis. The region of bone between the growth plate and the shaft (diaphysis) of a long bone.

MRI aka MR. Magnetic resonance imaging.

MVA (USA) aka Motor vehicle accident (USA), Road traffic accident or RTA (UK).

Non-accidental injury (NAI) aka Battered baby, Battered child, Child abuse. Euphemism for a deliberate assault and injury to a young child or infant.

Nursemaid's elbow (USA) aka Pulled elbow (UK).

Occipitomental radiograph of the face (OM) aka Water's projection. Radiograph of facial bones obtained with the axis of the X-ray beam directed between chin and occiput. A following number (eg OM30 or OM15) denotes the degree of angulation of the X-ray beam.

Odontoid peg aka the dens, or the peg of the axis (C2) vertebra.

Oedema (UK) aka Edema (USA).

OPG aka Orthopantomogram, OPT, Panoramic view. A tomographic device specifically designed to demonstrate the mandible and part of the maxilla.

Ossification. The process by which bone is formed. Most commonly bone forms from cartilage (eg a long bone). Less commonly bone forms from membrane (eg skull). Ossification can also occur in the soft tissues either as the result of haemorrhage following trauma or due to chronic inflammation.

Osteochondral fracture. Fracture involving a joint surface and the fracture fragment consists of a small piece of bone and cartilage. The cartilaginous component is invisible on the plain radiograph. Example: osteochondral fracture of the dome of the talus.

PA. Postero-anterior. Indicates the direction of the X-ray beam passing through the patient.

Paediatrics (UK) Pediatrics (USA).

Palmar. Relating to the palm of the hand (ie the ventral surface).

Periosteal new bone formation aka Periosteal reaction, subperiosteal new bone formation. Appearance of a thin white line along part of the shaft of a long bone which appears to be separated from the cortex by a small space. The periosteum is invisible on a radiograph, and the reaction (or new bone) is a layer of ossification deep to the invisible periosteum. The small space between the white line and the bone is due to elevation of the periosteum by blood, pus, or tumour. In the context of trauma a periosteal reaction is a normal healing response.

Physis. See Growth plate.

Plastic bowing fracture aka Plastic deformity, Bowing fracture. A type of long bone fracture occuring in children. The force is predominantly that of a longitudinal stress on an immature long bone. A series of microfractures occur, causing the bone to bend, adopting a smooth curve, with no obvious abnormality of the cortex. Most commonly occurring in the forearm bones; may also affect the tibia, the fibula, and the clavicle.

Radiographer (UK) aka Radiographic technician (USA) or Radiologic technologist (USA).

Radionuclide investigation. See: Isotope investigation.

Renal colic aka Ureteral colic, Ureteric colic.

RTA aka Road traffic accident (UK), Motor vehicle accident or MVA (USA).

Scaphoid bone (UK) aka Carpal navicular (USA).

Scintigraphy. See: Isotope investigation.

Sclerotic. Denotes a dense (white) line or area on a radiograph. May be at the periphery or cortex of a bone (eg the sclerotic appearance of maturing callus surrounding a healing fracture), or traversing the shaft of a bone (eg impacted fracture).

Glossary

Screening (UK) aka Fluoroscopy (UK, USA). Fluoroscopic screening. See: Fluoroscopy.

Skyline view aka Sunrise or Sunset view. A tangential radiograph of the knee which provides a supero-inferior view of the patella and of the patellofemoral joint.

Stress fracture aka Fatigue fracture, March fracture. A fracture resulting from minor but repeated injury to an otherwise normal and healthy bone.

Subluxation. The articular surfaces of adjacent bones maintain some contact; ie the joint surfaces are no longer congruous but contact has not been completely disrupted.

Sudeck's atrophy aka Reflex sympathetic dystrophy syndrome. Chronic persistent pain associated with severe localised reduction in bone density. Most commonly occurs as a result of trauma with or without a fracture.

Swimmer's view. A lateral projection used to show the cervicothoracic junction. The name derives from the patient's position (one arm fully extended, the other by the side), which simulates that of a swimmer doing either the back stroke or the crawl (freestyle).

Symphysis. A joint between adjacent bones lined by hyaline cartilage and stabilised by fibrocartilage and ligaments. Example: symphysis pubis.

Synchondrosis. The site of a persistent plate of cartilage between adjacent bones, at which little or no movement occurs. Example: zygomaticofrontal synchondrosis.

Technician (USA) aka Radiographer (UK), Radiographic Technician (USA), Radiologic Technologist (USA).

Tibial plafond. The distal articular surface of the tibia.

Trapezium bone (UK) aka Greater multangular (USA).

Trapezoid bone (UK) aka Lesser multangular (USA).

Triquetral bone aka Triquetrum.

Tuberosity. Any prominence on a bone to which a tendon or tendons are attached (eg tuberosity at the base of the fifth metatarsal).

Two Bone Rule. See description on page 146.

Valgus. An angular deformity at a joint or fracture site in which the distal bone (or bone fragment) is deviated away from the midline.

Varus. An angular deformity at a joint or fracture site in which the deviation of the distal bone (or bone fragment) is towards the midline.

Ventral. Relating to the anterior (flexor) aspect of the body or body part (eg a limb). See: Dorsal.

Vertical beam radiograph. Denotes the orientation of the X-ray beam with respect to the floor. The beam is at right angles to the floor.

View. aka Projection, Position, or Method. In the context of diagnostic radiology this refers to the position of the patient, or of the X-ray tube, when a radiographic exposure occurs. Examples: frontal view, lateral view.

Volar. Relating to the palm of the hand or the sole of the foot.

Well corticated. A term used to describe the appearance of the periphery of a bone (eg an accessory ossicle) where it is seen to have a dense smooth margin. This appearance contrasts with the incompletely corticated margin of a fracture fragment

Further reading:

Lee P, Hunter TB, Taljanovic M. Musculoskeletal Colloquialisms: How Did We Come Up with These Names? Radiographics 2004;24:1009–1027.

Index

Index

Index

Index

Test Yourself—answers

1. Galeazzi fracture dislocation, p. 146.
2. Stress (fatigue) fracture 3rd metatarsal, p. 299.
3. Normal. The widened space on the left side of the peg and the asymmetric alignment of the lateral masses on the right side are due to positional rotation of the neck, p. 182.
4. Isolated blow out fracture of the left orbit with a teardrop and haemorrhage (fluid level) in the maxillary antrum, pp. 64–67.
5. Apical oblique view of the shoulder, p. 76; posterior dislocation of the head of the humerus, p. 89.
6. Odontoid peg fracture, p. 188.
7. Apical oblique view of the shoulder; p. 76. (1) Anterior dislocation of the head of the humerus, p. 84. (2) Detached fragment medial to the head; (3) Hill–Sach's lesion, p. 85.
8. Bennett's fracture—dislocation of the thumb, p. 165.
9. Undisplaced fracture of the distal radius, p. 136.
10. Fat-fluid level in the suprapatellar bursa, p. 249; an intra-articular fracture is not evident on this single view, but is presumed to be present.
11. Supracondylar fracture with minimal posterior displacement, pp. 106–108.
12. Dislocations at the 4th and 5th carpometacarpal joints, pp. 156–157, 168.
13. Greenstick fracture of the distal radius, pp. 18–19.
14. Normal OM radiograph, pp. 55, 60–61.
15. Avulsion of the apophysis of the right anterior inferior iliac spine (AIIS), pp. 223, 236–237.
16. Fractures of the C6 and C7 spinous processes, pp. 192.
17. Fracture of the lateral tibial plateau, pp. 250–253.
18. Central dislocation/displacement of the right femoral head. Acetabular fracture, pp. 219, 240.
19. The important finding: fracture through the neck of the talus, p. 282.
20. Normal Lisfranc joints and normal tarsal bones, pp. 294–297, 303.
21. Normal apophysis at the base of 5th metatarsal, p. 298; multicentric ossification is also normal, p. 305.
22. Dislocated head of the radius, pp. 104, 112.
23. Subluxation at the acromioclavicular joint. Also, suspect a tear of the coracoclavicular ligaments, pp. 86–87.
24. Fracture involving the volar plate, and a mallet finger fracture, pp. 154, 159, 161.
25. Fracture of the calcaneum: abnormal Bohler's angle, pp. 277–279.
26. Segond fracture, p. 259.
27. (1) Forward subluxation of C4 on C5 vertebra, p. 193; (2) fracture of the odontoid peg, pp. 188–189.
28. Lisfranc-subluxation at the base of the 2nd metatarsal, pp. 295–297, 302–303.